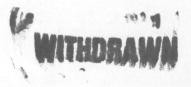
THE FIRST YEAR®

Parkinson's Disease

An Essential Guide for the Newly Diagnosed

JACKIE HUNT CHRISTENSEN was diagnosed with Parkinson's disease in 1998 at the age of thirty-four and has been active in the Parkinson Association of Minnesota, the Parkinson's Action Network, and the Young-Onset Parkinson Network of the National Parkinson Foundation ever since. Retired from her food safety work at the Institute for Agriculture and Trade Policy (IATP), Christensen lives in Minneapolis with her husband and two sons, where she continues to do volunteer work on environmental health issues.

THE COMPLETE FIRST YEAR® SERIES

The First Year—Type 2 Diabetes by Gretchen Becker

The First Year—IBS by Heather Van Vorous

The First Year—Hepatitis C by Cara Bruce and Lisa Montanarelli

The First Year—Fibroids by Johanna Skilling

The First Year—Hepatitis B by William Finley Green

The First Year—Crohn's Disease and Ulcerative Colitis by Jill Sklar

The First Year—Multiple Sclerosis by Margaret Blackstone

The First Year—Hypothyroidism by Maureen Pratt

The First Year—Fibromyalgia by Claudia Craig Marek

The First Year—HIV by Brett Grodeck

The First Year—Lupus by Nancy Hangar

The First Year—Scleroderma by Karen Gottesman

The First Year—Prostate Cancer by Christopher Lukas

FORTHCOMING

The First Year—Rheumatoid Arthritis by M.E.A. McNeil

THE FIRST YEAR®

Parkinson's Disease

An Essential Guide for the Newly Diagnosed

Jackie Hunt Christensen

Foreword by Paul J. Tuite, MD

MARLOWE & COMPANY ▪ NEW YORK

THE FIRST YEAR® — PARKINSON'S DISEASE:
An Essential Guide for the Newly Diagnosed
Copyright © 2005 by Jackie Hunt Christensen
Foreword copyright © 2005 by Paul J. Tuite, MD

Published by
Marlowe & Company
An Imprint of Avalon Publishing Group Incorporated
245 West 17th Street, 11th Floor
New York, NY 10011

AVALON
publishing group incorporated

The First Year® and A Patient-Expert Walks You Through Everything
You Need to Learn and Do® are trademarks of
the Avalon Publishing Group.

Library of Congress Control Number: 2005932147
ISBN: 1-56924-372-7
ISBN-13: 978-1-56924-372-5

9 8 7 6 5 4 3 2

Designed by Pauline Neuwirth,
  Neuwirth and Associates, Inc.

Printed in the United States of America

For Paul:
You are the friend of my days,
the lover of my nights, and
the father of my children.
I love you truly, madly, deeply.
Thank you for walking with me
and holding my hand through
yet another FOG.

Contents

Foreword

by Paul J. Tuite, MD

PARKINSON'S DISEASE is a degenerative disorder that is associated with the loss of brain cells that produce the chemical dopamine. A decreasing level of dopamine in the brain leads to the multitude of motor symptoms that manifest as slowness, tremor, stiffness, and altered posture. As well, a variety of other features appear over time, which reflect the involvement of additional systems of the body. In essence, Parkinson's disease is an insidious condition that begins to impact nearly all facets of life in addition to the obvious motor changes. Hence, with disease progression comes increasing problems. Fortunately, there is help out there for those with Parkinson's disease—from family members, the health-care team, patient support and advocacy groups, and an assortment of other individuals. It is my and Jackie Christensen's hope that this book will also prove useful.

Jackie has spent much of her professional career enhancing awareness of environmental issues and implementing change to make this a healthier world. Since developing Parkinson's disease, she has faced challenges to make a change in the world as it views this condition, which parallels the difficulties she faced to get people to notice the environment. Specifically, as a young person with Parkinson's disease, she has had to deal with ignorance about a condition that can affect those as young as thirty or forty; ambivalence about environmental factors that may play a role in disease causation; and passivity regarding conventional, novel, and alternative therapies. Furthermore, she and others have faced numerous roadblocks that affect the search for better treatments and potential cures.

It is Jackie's wish, as well as my own, that politicians, physicians, scientists, and the numerous Parkinson's disease organizations will align their priorities and efforts to work together for a cure. This book is an attempt to provide a guide to others who are impacted by Parkinson's disease and to provide signposts to remind us that we are not alone on this path and there is help. One first step in this process is learning how to grab hold of life after first hearing the words "You have Parkinson's disease." For some, hope comes through reading, thinking, and reflecting upon the words of someone like Jackie; however, for others, reading may be frustrating and overwhelming. If that is the case, set the book down for a while, but remember it is there like a trusty friend who can be turned to when needed.

PAUL TUITE, MD, is associate professor of neurology at the University of Minnesota and director of the Parkinson's Disease and Movement Disorders Clinic at the University of Minnesota Medical Center. He lives with his wife, Marilee, in Minneapolis.

Introduction

I WANT to begin by expressing my admiration for you, as a newly diagnosed or recently diagnosed person with Parkinson's disease, for having the courage to learn more about this intrusion into your life. Parkinson's disease will affect how you live your life from now until a cure is found or you pass away. However, I believe that coping with it is much easier if you remember that you are not your disease; you are the same person you have always been, but now always accompanied by an uninvited guest who will monopolize and control your life as much as you let it.

Knowledge is power

Parkinson's disease (PD) is the second most prevalent degenerative neurological disease in America, after Alzheimer's disease. Somewhere between one million and one-and-a-half million people have been diagnosed with Parkinson's, and certainly many more have symptoms but have not been told by a doctor that they have the disease. If you have been diagnosed with Parkinson's disease, you are in some august company: Muhammad Ali,

Janet Reno, and Michael J. Fox, to name a few famous people currently living with PD, too. As I write this, Pope John Paul II has just recently passed away from complications of Parkinson's disease. The internationally renowned painter, Salvador Dali; Chinese leader Teng Hsiao-p'ing; General Douglas MacArthur; and actor Jim Backus, who played Thurston Howell on *Gilligan's Island* and provided the voice for the cartoon character Mr. Magoo, all had PD. The attention brought to the disease by celebrities has definitely helped to raise awareness and money for research. Chances are, you don't have the resources or disposable income that they do, but by being an informed, assertive patient, you can have excellent care and live a full life while waiting for a cure to be found. Researchers say they are very close. In the meantime, may this book help you cope.

The more that you learn about PD, the better equipped you will be to catch new developments in your disease early and get treatment, protect yourself from complications, make sure you are getting the care that is best for you, and improve your overall quality of life.

How my journey with Parkinson's disease began

My personal journey with Parkinson's disease began shortly after my son Bennett was born in 1996. I had gone back to my job as director of the Food Safety Project at the Institute for Agriculture and Trade Policy six weeks after his birth. This position involved doing a great deal of online research about environmental contaminants in food, writing educational materials, organizing conference calls and meetings—in short, a lot of sitting and typing. I quickly discovered that when I tried to type, my ring finger and pinkie on my left hand did not want to strike the intended keys. I assumed that it was carpal tunnel syndrome and had my workspace's ergonomics checked. I saw an orthopedist, who said it wasn't carpal tunnel but offered no other suggestions. I was relieved to hear that my hand seemed physically sound, but that did not alleviate my symptoms. In addition to the stubborn fingers, I sometimes had a tremor in my thumb. My left hand was often much colder than the right and had a pins-and-needles sensation that was very disconcerting.

The next symptoms I noticed were pain and extreme tightness in my left shoulder. I couldn't lift my arm above my head, and the movements I could make with it felt mechanical. My shoulder felt like a set of gears that needed a lube job. One evening as I was watering my flower garden, I noticed that my left arm was curled up at my side rather than swinging as I walked. After that, I kept track of my arm's position. It always seemed to end up in that curled position. Also, the hamstring in my left leg seemed perpetually taut, despite nightly yoga stretches.

My primary physician treated my hand, shoulder, and leg as separate problems, despite my feeling that they were all connected. She referred me to Neurologist #1, who had a bad case of "compassion fatigue." I had had one CT scan of my head performed, yet he told me that he didn't know what was wrong with me and there were no more tests that could be done. (I know now that this was absolutely untrue.) He seemed annoyed when I began to cry (What did he expect? I was a sleep-deprived mother of a five-year-old and an eight-month-old and was working full-time. I had just been diagnosed with Crohn's disease, a very painful gastrointestinal condition, and was taking large amounts of prednisone, a powerful steroid notorious for making people very emotional.).

I had been doing some research online about my symptoms. Ironically, I had come across Parkinson's disease, but assumed, as so many people do, that it was only an "old person's disease." My symptoms were also indicative of multiple sclerosis, so I asked the doctor whether that could be my problem.

"If that's what you want me to write down, I will," he barked.

"Of course not!" I replied, shocked and appalled at his lack of professionalism. "I just want to know what's wrong with me! I don't WANT to have anything." My only consolation in all this was that my husband was there with me, so I had a witness. Nevertheless, I waited two or three months to get a second opinion and vowed never to see that doctor again under any circumstances.

Neurologist #2 came right out and told me to see a psychiatrist. This doctor makes me feel extremely lucky to be living with PD now, instead of as recently as fifty years ago. Back then, doctors like him would have written a Valium prescription, scheduled a hysterectomy, and if that didn't do the trick, put me in an institution.

It took visits to another orthopedist, a neurosurgeon (who told me that I have two mildly herniated discs in my spine that were not responsible for my symptoms), a physiatrist, and a physical therapist before Neurologist #3 came up with the potential diagnosis of "hemiparkinsonism" ("hemi-" just means one-half or one-sided). I reacted with shock and surprise. "At least you're not crazy," he said.

He gave me a prescription for Sinemet, saying, "If this helps, then we assume it is Parkinson's disease." He explained that there was not (and still is not) a test for diagnosing PD that can be done on living patients. The Sinemet helped almost immediately, and I have been on it ever since.

Dealing with the diagnosis

I believe that in the final analysis people deal with the diagnosis of a chronic illness in one of two ways:

- ○ They seek and are relieved to finally have a diagnosis and believe, now that the problem has been identified, they can face it and get on with their lives. These people are more likely to take an active role in their treatment from the get-go and do all they can to learn about the disease and treatment options.
- ○ They believe that as long as there is no diagnosis, they can hold on to the hope that it is just a virus or a pulled muscle or stress—some condition that will go away on its own. Upon receiving a diagnosis of Parkinson's disease, people in this category are more likely to withdraw into a depression and may ignore important symptoms or delay seeing a doctor, due to their refusal to accept that they have a chronic illness.

Of course, most circumstances in life are not that cut and dried. On average, most people who are ultimately diagnosed with Parkinson's disease see three or four doctors before the diagnosis is confirmed. Along the way, you can easily become discouraged and wonder if you are crazy.

One of the complicating factors in your quest for answers is the lack of a definitive diagnostic test to confirm a PD diagnosis. Another factor is the existence of some subtypes within Parkinson's disease as well as other degenerative disorders that resemble PD. These conditions often result in additional visits to more doctors and make it especially challenging to write an all-encompassing guide for newly diagnosed individuals.

The fact that you are reading this book indicates that you are willing to dip your toe into the pool of knowledge about Parkinson's disease. I want you to know that all of us with PD have hours or days when we retreat into denial; that is normal.

However, since that awful expedition through the nearly impassable river of confusion that has been my experience with much of our health-care system, I came out on the other side. I have survived and have met amazing, inspiring people in my support group and at conferences whom I would never have met if I had not developed PD. I have hobbies now, which I didn't have before. I go fishing; I make beaded jewelry and do other crafts; I am now exploring the soothing world of watercolor painting. (It seems as if the more Parkinson's disease affects my speaking voice, the more time I spend trying to express myself through new and varied creative projects.) And as much as I have cried and yelled and sworn out of anger and frustration with this disease (and will do so again, many more times), I have come to recognize a strength in myself that I didn't know was there. You have it, too. It takes inner strength, fortitude, chutzpah, whatever you want to call it, to face each day.

To me, our individual experiences with Parkinson's disease seem rather like the forced relocation experienced by Native Americans as their nations were uprooted. What we all share is the invasion of our bodies by an unin-vited guest called Parkinson's disease, which is colonizing our brain, forc-ing us to leave the familiar surroundings of daily life as we have known it. We are not sure where we are going or what we will find when we get there. Some of us will find ourselves ambushed by debilitating symptoms that very quickly render us incapable of work. Others make the journey very slowly, with only fairly minor inconveniences. But there is one circumstance over which we do have control: our attitude toward our "invader."

My hopes for you

I want this book to help other newly diagnosed people avoid feeling as this person did.

> Even though no two cases are alike, it would be nice to have someone say, 'This is what you can probably expect from your future." Is this as good as it gets or is there some positive thing I can hang my hat on? —MATT, *diagnosed at 49*

Yes, Matt, there can be many positive changes in your life, if you have the right attitude. It is my hope that this book will help you to get in touch with the "warrior" part of you that will struggle to be informed, stall the advance of the disease with any means with which you are comfortable, and embrace the surprising blessings that can also accompany PD. I hope that by the time you finish reading, you will feel hopeful, connected to a larger whole, and inspired to find the joy in your life each and every day.

The limitations of this book

I will not prescribe treatment for your Parkinson's disease. I am not a health professional; therefore, I cannot prescribe treatment for you or tell you what is best for your particular form of Parkinson's disease. I see my task as presenting the range of options available as I am writing this (fall 2004 through spring 2005), so that you can discuss them with your family and physician. I am not a scientist, and I suspect that many of you are not either, so my aim is to keep the content of the book fairly basic and to direct you to other resources for highly detailed or technical information.

This book cannot tell you how Parkinson's disease will affect you specifically, nor can it predict how your disease will progress. This is one of the mixed blessings of having PD—if you see someone with extreme tremors or slowness of movement, you can take heart in knowing that there is no guarantee that you will experience those symptoms to that degree. On the other hand, you might.

I cannot possibly cover every treatment or test, because we are living in an age where new research is being done every day to find the cause(s) and cure for PD and to develop treatments to help us cope until a cure is available. Because I am not a doctor or a scientist, I have relied on their advice and on research that has been published in peer-reviewed journals or is reported in government publications or by national PD groups.

Unless I am citing a particular physician as a reference for a specific piece of information, I will not identify doctors or health practitioners by name. I will give you the contact information for national or regional organizations that can help you to find a health-care provider in your area.

Finally, this book will probably not be an "easy read," one that you breeze through in a day. The issues that Parkinson's disease forces you to address are emotional, complex, and ongoing. I will not sugarcoat the information that I present. I am stating the technical/factual information as matter-of-factly as possible; these are the "Learning" sections of the book. The "Living" sections include quotes and anecdotes from other people with Parkinson's or from their care partners who have shared some of their feelings about their experiences.

A *note about "time"*

"Day 1" of your Parkinson's disease almost certainly occurred years ago. Most people don't notice symptoms until 60 to 80 percent of their dopamine-producing neurons are gone, and it may take months or years longer to receive a diagnosis. Please keep this in mind as you read this book. Because of the unique way that Parkinson's disease affects each person, think of the chronology as a framework for presenting the information, rather than as a timeline. Although *The First Year—Parkinson's Disease* is ostensibly about your first year after diagnosis, there is information here that will benefit you at any stage of your illness, such as anecdotes about waiting to be diagnosed and what you might expect from the condition years down the line. I will consider this book a success if I can help every person with PD who reads it come away with at least one new piece of information, a new way of coping with some aspect of the disease, a better understanding of it, or an idea of your own to help others with Parkinson's disease.

Yours in the struggle to find the cause and cure,
JACKIE HUNT CHRISTENSEN

THE FIRST YEAR®

Parkinson's Disease

An Essential Guide for the Newly Diagnosed

What Exactly Is Parkinson's Disease?

YOU HAVE been told by a health-care provider that you have Parkinson's disease, and you probably have a lot of questions, such as, "What exactly is Parkinson's disease?" "How does it affect my body?" "Will it kill me?" "I don't shake; how can I have Parkinson's?"

Parkinson's disease defined

Parkinson's disease (which, from now on, I will generally refer to as PD or just "Parkinson's") is named after James Parkinson, who in 1817 wrote about the condition he called "the shaking palsy." It is a chronic, progressive neurological disease that affects the **substantia nigra's** ability to produce **dopamine**. In other words, the disease affects the part of your brain that makes a chemical messenger (dopamine) that helps tell your muscles what to do. This disease does not go away and will get worse over time. That is not very uplifting news, but after all, you are reading this book to find out what you might be able to expect. Throughout this book, I will refer to those of us with Parkinson's disease as "**Parkies.**" I use the term because it is shorter, and I find it much less pretentious than the alternatively used "**parkinsonian**." I apologize in advance if you find this offensive. We've got to have a sense of humor or we'll never get through this!

Generally, by the time PD is diagnosed, 60 to 80 percent of the dopamine-producing cells in your brain, known as **dopaminergic neurons**, are no longer functioning. This means that you have had the disease for years without knowing it. For most people, it will be several more years before you are seriously debilitated by the disease, and who knows what might happen between now and then. There is a considerable amount of research being done to find the cause and cure for Parkinson's, and new therapies are becoming available.

While Parkinson's is an "equal-opportunity" disease that hits men and women from all ethnic backgrounds and socioeconomic levels in all parts of the country, it also affects each person differently. Even then, it is essentially a new disease every day. No one can claim that dealing with Parkinson's disease is boring!

Some facts about Parkinson's disease

Although history shows that Parkinson's disease has been around for thousands of years, it may amaze you how much is not known about it. Here is some of the information that we do have:

> The only predictable thing about this disease is that it is unpredictable. —RICHARD KRAMER, *who was diagnosed with Parkinson's disease at age 36*

- O It is not contagious.
- O It will get worse over time and will not go away on its own.
- O There is no known cause or cure.
- O Parkinson's disease itself is not fatal. It's the complications that may occur with the disease that can lead to death.
- O More than one million Americans are affected. (Exact numbers are uncertain, because PD can be difficult to diagnose and there is no national registry to keep track.)
- O Parkinson's disease is the second most common degenerative neurological disease in America (Alzheimer's disease is first), and there are

more people with PD than the combined number of cases of amyotrophic lateral sclerosis (ALS, also known as Lou Gehrig's disease), multiple sclerosis, muscular dystrophy, and myasthenia gravis.[1]

○ The majority—at least 60 percent—of people who develop Parkinson's disease are age fifty-five or older when diagnosed.

○ The combined direct and indirect costs of Parkinson's disease, including treatment, Social Security payments, and lost income from inability to work, are estimated to be more than $66 million per day in the United States alone.[2]

○ A new case of Parkinson's disease is diagnosed about every nine minutes.[3]

○ Slightly more men are affected than women.

○ Rates of PD are higher in the Midwestern farming states of Minnesota, Iowa, North and South Dakota, and Nebraska.[4]

○ The average age of onset is sixty years.

○ Most cases are not hereditary.

○ The number of cases and the incidence rate of PD vary from country to country, and possibly, among different ethnic groups. There is conflicting information about whether Caucasians have higher rates of PD than African Americans and Asian Americans.[5]

Hallmarks of Parkinson's disease

There are four signs that physicians consider when making a diagnosis of Parkinson's disease. ("Signs" are what the doctors observe; "symptoms" are what we experience.) In nearly all cases of PD, the patient will experience symptoms on one side of the body when they are first diagnosed. Later, symptoms will affect both sides of the body.

Tremor

Tremors are the most obvious symptom, so if you don't have tremors or other symptoms that are more pronounced, you may not get diagnosed right away. This was certainly true for me, and it seems fairly common in young-onset PD cases where tremor was not the primary symptom.

Shaking, or tremor, is a rhythmical involuntary movement that is the first symptom noted in 50 percent of Parkinson's cases. It is the symptom that most people associate with Parkinson's disease, but many of us never have a tremor. When a tremor is present, it typically occurs in your hand or leg when that limb is not moving or is at rest (thus, it is called a **resting tremor**.) At times the tremor may be also present when you are engaged in an activity. That is called an **action tremor** and does not usually occur early in the disease. Some people report an internal tremor that may not be visible to others.

Your jaw may be affected, but generally, the head and the voice are not affected in PD. Head and voice tremors are common in **essential tremor (ET)**. The classic movie actress Katharine Hepburn had ET. Sometimes separating the diagnosis of PD and ET is challenging because it is possible to have both. As with PD, the individuals who have ET develop other motor symptoms in addition to tremor over time. Unfortunately, it may take months to years before a physician can determine whether a person has one or both conditions.

Finally, although by definition tremors are rhythmical, the severity of tremor can change under different circumstances, such as stress, excitement, or anticipation. For example, you might be at a party where you feel like you are relaxed and at ease, yet your thumb or foot may begin twitching because you are excited to be there.

Many people say that their tremor started with a back-and-forth movement of the thumb and forefinger. Doctors refer to this as "pill-rolling." Tremors usually stop when we are asleep. Approximately 15 percent of people with PD don't experience tremors at all.[6] If you are one of those people, as I have been, there will be those who doubt your diagnosis. They have a lot to learn.

MUSCLE RIGIDITY

All muscles have an "opposing muscle." Our muscles move smoothly when one muscle in the pair contracts while its counterpart relaxes. The **rigidity** associated with PD occurs because the natural give-and-take relationship that our muscles normally have has been disturbed. In the case of PD, the opposing muscle does not relax normally. This resistance to movement is the rigidity we feel. It can occur in your neck and back, arms, or legs. It may be only one side of your body. If your doctor refers to your condition as **hemiparkinsonism,** she or he merely means that one side of your body is affected.

This stiffness is different than the feeling that comes with arthritis or age. At times I feel like a scarecrow, with my head like a feedbag of sawdust perched precariously on a broom-handle spine. Before my diagnosis, I remember being asked if I had been in a car accident because my upper body was so tense that I could hardly turn my head.

There are two types of rigidity related to PD. One is called **lead pipe rigidity,** because your body's muscles resist movement and getting them to move is like trying to bend a lead pipe.[7] The other is called **cogwheel rigidity** because of the jerky motion caused by an underlying tremor that occurs when your arm or leg is moved. Regardless of the semantics, rigidity affects fluid (smooth, graceful) movements and can cause pain. Rigidity can be treated with physical therapies, such as yoga or tai chi, with medication, or both approaches.

SLOWNESS OF MOVEMENT

The clinical term for slowness of movement is **bradykinesia,** and it is extremely frustrating, especially for high-strung, impatient people like me. You may find that your problem is not that you are unable to do the activities you have always done; it just takes much longer. You will have to think about movements that used to be effortless. This requires more concentration, which can be stressful. This leads to more fatigue.

For example, repetitive movements such as brushing teeth will become difficult. For some reason, so-called automatic movements, or **reflexes,** are more affected than learned movements. Doing two or more things at a time will become problematic—no more walking and chewing gum.

With time, people with Parkinson's may have trouble initiating a movement or beginning to speak. This is called **start hesitancy,** or some call it **freezing** (even those who live outside of Minnesota). Freezing occurs because of problems implementing learned motor programs. The idea to do an activity just does not quite make it into the action/implementation part of the brain, and you will need to figure out ways to overcome or work around these mental blocks. Sometimes you can use visual or auditory cues to get yourself going. Some people find the use of striped patterns on the floor helpful in getting started walking; others step over a cane that has been laid flat on the floor, march in place, or use tapping sounds in their head to get going.

A condition known as **blepharospasm,** which involves involuntary changes or slowness in blinking, can cause dry eyes. Slowed swallowing reflexes, combined with excess saliva, can cause choking. Your reflexes may not kick in quickly enough to get your hands out in front of you if you fall. Poor balance will cause a fall, and our inability to react in time to break our fall can lead to broken bones.

POOR BALANCE

You may find yourself tripping or stumbling often. Perhaps you feel as though you are about to tip over backward. Sometimes scientific journals call this **postural instability**. You will have to think twice about using ladders or scaffolding. These balance problems may occur because the brain in Parkinson's disease does not quite respond as quickly to changes in posture, and the sensory information sent to the brain may be faulty. Unfortunately, balance impairment remains poorly understood and treatment is still being explored in the laboratories of kinesiologists, physical therapists, and engineers.

When two of the above four signs are present, your doctor will consider Parkinson's disease as a diagnosis. Some PD information sources list five signs, the fifth being **akinesia**—absence of movement. For example, you may have noticed that one of your arms does not swing when you walk. When five signs are considered, the presence of three of the five indicates PD as the likely diagnosis.

Not only does PD affect everyone differently, but it will also affect you differently each day—perhaps even each hour! This is a mixed blessing, because it will allow you to have moments when you can forget that you have a chronic illness, but it can also make it difficult to qualify for disability, supplemental Social Security, or other benefits.

IN A SENTENCE:

> *Doctors look for four signs of Parkinson's disease when they are making a diagnosis, but not everyone will experience all of them.*

Techniques Doctors Use to Diagnose PD

A **DIAGNOSIS** of Parkinson's disease is a diagnosis of exclusion. Physicians order tests to eliminate other possibilities: a brain tumor, **Wilson's disease, multiple sclerosis,** and other conditions. In determining that you do not have any of those conditions, your doctor probably ran several, if not all, of the tests described below.

Tests used to exclude other diseases

The goal of these tests is literally to see what is going on inside your head. Keep in mind that these procedures are tools, not a litmus test that can verify your disease.

CAT SCAN

CAT scan (also known as a CT scan) stands for "computerized axial tomography." It is an imaging test (one that produces pictures) that uses a form of radiation to get a three-dimensional view of your head, neck, or whatever part of the body is scanned. It's generally used to detect bleeding or bone problems. Like an X-ray, it is painless and relatively quick. The procedure is performed by a technician, who gives the results to a radiologist. The radiologist will then discuss the results with your doctor.

CAT scans are not useful in distinguishing between Parkinson's disease and other **degenerative** parkinsonian conditions that may resemble PD, such as **progressive supranuclear palsy** (also known as **PSP)** or **multiple system atrophy (MSA)**. PSP and MSA belong to the parkinsonian family and some classify them in a category of disorders called **Parkinson's Plus (PD+).** (You will read more about those conditions in Day 3.)

MRI

Magnetic resonance imaging (MRI) is a technology that uses magnetic fields to get two- or three-dimensional "pictures" of part of your body.[8] For this test, you lie on a platform that slides you into a tube or tunnel inside a large "box." You have to remain still for several periods of a few minutes at a time. A loud tapping sound is produced as the waves of energy reflect back to your body. You may be offered earplugs to lessen the noise. If you are claustrophobic, you may be offered a mild sedative to assure that you do not move during the test. Sometimes a contrast dye will be injected prior to scanning to improve the doctor's ability to see abnormalities if they are present. For **parkinsonism**, a brain MRI would be performed to rule out multiple sclerosis and other disorders such as **normal pressure hydrocephalus.**

The use of MRI and CT scans is presently limited by their ability to detect structural changes in the brain. Early on in the course of PSP or MSA, selective and local changes are not visible with MRI and may never been seen due to the limitations of the technology in detecting microscopic changes.

PET AND SPECT SCANS

PET scans (positron emission tomography) and **SPECT scans (single photon emission commuted computed tomography)** are imaging technologies that employ radioactive compounds and may be useful for distinguishing Parkinson's from the symptoms of normal aging. However, the technologies remain experimental, very expensive, and are not widely available. For the most part, these scans are being used to test for PD+ if someone is not getting relief from Sinemet or if the person's disease is progressing quite rapidly.

Other tests that might be done

In his book *Parkinson's Disease: The Way Forward*, British author and physician Geoffrey Leader encourages his PD patients to undergo a number of tests that I find quite interesting but are not routinely conducted in the United States.[9] These include blood analysis of your immune system; electrolytes; liver and kidney function; thyroid levels; and mercury. Dr. Leader also recommends sweat or blood tests for toxic metals and pesticides. To date, no published data has demonstrated a clear relationship between an abnormality found in these laboratory tests and someone who has been diagnosed with PD.

Because the symptoms of Parkinson's disease tend to become apparent gradually, it can be difficult to diagnose in the early stages. Sometimes a patient may not have **idiopathic Parkinson's disease** but will have some other form of parkinsonism. The Michael J. Fox Foundation for Parkinson's Research estimates that 20 percent of PD patients are misdiagnosed.[10]

Unlike diabetes or cancer, there isn't a test that can be performed to definitively confirm a PD diagnosis while you are alive. When you are dead, doctors can examine the substantia nigra in your brain, but that doesn't really do you any good. Nonetheless, at each visit with your health-care provider, you will be evaluated to confirm your diagnosis as well as to track the progression of the disease. (I know that right now you are thinking, "Maybe the doctor was wrong. I don't have Parkinson's. It was a mistake and I have something that can be cured with a pill or an operation! Chances are, if you had something that was readily curable, it would have been identified by now.)

Researchers at the **National Institutes of Health (NIH)** and others are working to find a **biomarker,** some part of your body—blood, urine, or spinal fluid, for example—that could be tested when you first notice a problem. In January 2005, pharmaceutical giant Pfizer Inc. announced that its researchers had conducted voice testing and found that very subtle voice changes that are not perceptible to the human ear begin in PD patients years before other symptoms manifest themselves. Pfizer does not plan to market this seven-minute test but has used it successfully in their laboratories to detect schizophrenia and depression.[11]

Testing does not stop once you have been given a PD diagnosis; it merely changes. There are a number of physical tasks that your doctor will ask you to perform to track the progression of your disease and to identify new symptoms that may require treatment. You may be asked to do some of these tests each time you see your doctor. Others may be conducted less frequently.

Tests to evaluate the progression of your disease

There are several tests your doctor will use to see how and at what rate your condition is progressing.

DO THE HOKEY-POKEY—THE NEUROLOGICAL EXAM

I refer to this exam as "doing the hokey-pokey" or "doing party tricks," because whenever I'm asked to do these things, I feel like a child at a birthday party. If I listen closely and do exactly as I'm told, I'll get a prize, and if I screw up, I'll be humiliated. I have yet to win a prize, unless a new prescription counts. It also reminds me of the hokey-pokey, because it involves shaking various limbs as instructed. Having a sense of humor about it helps, because from now on your health-care provider will probably make you perform at least some of these tasks.

Variations on patty-cake

You will sit facing the doctor, and she will ask you to use your index finger to touch her finger and then touch your nose. She will have you continue this process as she moves her finger around. She will ask you to do this as quickly as you can, watching to see how accurate your movements are. This test assesses how well your **cerebellum,** a part of your brain that is essential for fine-motor activity and balance, is functioning.

Next you will be asked to touch each finger to the thumb of the same hand as quickly as you can. This test will be done on both hands. This evaluates motor speed in attempt to track bradykinesia.

Another part of the test involves resting your hands on your thighs. You will be asked to turn your hand over sideways—palm up to palm down—on your thigh with one hand then the other.

Playing footsie

Think of it as practice for flirting with your partner or a potential love interest. The doctor will ask you to take the heel of one foot and run it down along the shin of the other. Then you will do the other side. (When you get home, you can demonstrate on your mate.) This is another test to measure coordination.

Musical chairs

Or if you prefer, "Pretend you are a high-fashion model." Your doctor will ask you to get up from your chair, walk across the room or down a hallway, turn around, and walk back toward him. He will be observing your balance, posture, speed, and sense of direction, as well as whether or not your arms move while you walk. The doctor will be there to catch you if you should trip or fall.

Toeing the line

As if you were performing a sobriety test, you will be asked to walk in a straight line, putting the heel of one foot directly in front of the toe of the other.

By the time you have performed all of these movements, you may wish that you could pretend that your doctor is a piñata, but do try to keep in mind that these tests are the best way to monitor how your disease is affecting your body.

EVALUATING STAGES OF PD

Once Parkinson's disease is diagnosed, your physician may periodically evaluate the progression of your disease by using assessment instruments such as the **Hoehn & Yahr Scale** and/or the **Universal Parkinson's Disease Rating Scale (UPDRS)**. (See Appendix for a copy of the UPDRS.)

The Hoehn & Yahr scale splits PD into six stages:

Stage Zero
1. No visible symptoms of Parkinson's disease

Stage One
1. Signs and symptoms on one side only
2. Symptoms mild
3. Symptoms inconvenient but not disabling
4. Usually presents with tremor of one limb

  5. Family/friends have noticed changes in posture, walking, facial expression

Stage Two
  1. Symptoms bilateral (on both sides of the body)
  2. Symptoms cause minimal disability
  3. Posture and gait (walking) affected

Stage Three
  1. Movements are significantly slowed
  2. Early impairment of equilibrium (balance) with walking or rising to stand
  3. Overall state of dysfunction is moderately severe

Stage Four
  1. Symptoms are severely disabling
  2. Still able to do limited walking
  3. Rigidity and slowness become more prominent symptom
  4. No longer able to live alone
  5. Tremor may lessen

Stage Five
  1. Onset of cachexia (a state of malnutrition and wasting)
  2. Patient has become a complete invalid
  3. Unable to stand or walk
  4. Requires constant nursing care

This scale is based on a modified version of one that was developed prior to the widespread availability of Sinemet.[12] Your doctor may or may not use this tool to measure the progress of your disease.

There is a "quality of life" scale that is more suited to helping you to evaluate the ways in which the disease is affecting your life. This is helpful in that you can seek more targeted assistance, should you need it. For example, you track the number of days during a week that you have trouble with a particular activity. The areas of the scale include mobility; **activities of daily living (ADL)**, such as getting dressed and brushing your teeth; emotional state; cognitive function; social support (status of your relationship with your care partner, family, etc.); and bodily functions.

Here is a slightly modified copy of the Parkinson's Disease Quality of Life Scale (PDQ-39):

How often in the last three months have you had trouble with:	Always	Most days	2–3 days/ week	Rarely	Never
Stiffness					
Feeling generally unwell					
Feeling that you are no longer able to do your hobbies					
Feeling tense					
Feeling insecure about yourself because of your physical condition					
Shaking of your hand(s)					
Feeling fatigued, worn out or having no energy					
Difficulties with sports or other physically active leisure activities					
Clumsiness					
Feeling embarrassed about your PD					
Shuffling your feet when you walk					
Having to postpone or cancel social activities because of your PD					
Feelings of extreme exhaustion					
Difficulties turning around while walking					
Fear of possible progression of your PD					
Handwriting					
Feeling less able to go on vacation or travel because of your PD					
Feeling insecure about yourself around others					
Difficulty getting a good night's sleep					
"On/off" periods					
Difficulty accepting/coming to terms with your illness					
Difficulty talking					
Difficulty signing your name in public					
Difficulty walking					
Drooling					
Feeling depressed or discouraged					
Frequent urination or wetting yourself					

How often in the last three months have you had trouble with:	Always	Most days	2–3 days/ week	Rarely	Never
Difficulty sitting still for long periods					
Difficulties driving					
Sudden extreme movements					
Difficulty concentrating					
Difficulty getting up from a chair/ sitting position					
Constipation					
Memory problems					
Difficulty turning in bed					
Sexual dysfunction or worry that PD is affecting your sex life					
Feeling worried about the possible consequences of an operation connected with your PD					
Did you need help completing this questionnaire	YES		NO		

"Stage THIS!"

Whatever you do, do not let these scales and surveys become an obsession! They are tools to help you and your doctor determine your course of treatment. If you find yourself worrying about how you have scored or the stage at which your physician gauged your PD, use it as an opportunity to work through your feelings about it.

Make a list of activities that are becoming more difficult. Make a parallel list of at least two related activities that you can still do. (What is important here is not the product, it is the process, so you do not need to be able to read your lists. If writing or typing is one of those things giving you trouble, you could use a tape recorder if you like. Or simply say the list items aloud to yourself.)

Here is an example:

I am having trouble . . .	But I can still . . . and . . .
Tying my shoes	Choose the shoes I want to wear and put them on myself if I buy ones that do not require shoelaces
Writing with a ballpoint pen	Use a pen with a large rubber grip; type on my computer; doodle on a piece of paper

To really get rid of some frustration, when you are sick of making lists, you can tear the pages into pieces or feed them into a shredder. If you made a recording, you can erase it. Parkinson's disease is difficult enough to deal with; we do not need to add to our burden by loading ourselves up with emotional baggage.

IN A SENTENCE:

> *There are a number of tests that your health-care provider will use to diagnose Parkinson's disease as well as track the efficacy of any medications you are taking and the progression of your illness.*

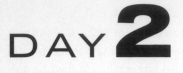

DAY 2

living

Early Symptoms of PD

IN ADDITION to the four primary signs that doctors use to classify your condition as Parkinson's disease, there are many other symptoms that you may in fact experience first.

Mood and personality changes/ cognitive difficulties

There are a variety of behavioral changes that may occur in PD, including **depression** and **anxiety.** One recent study found that people who are anxious or depressed and have a pessimistic outlook on life have an increased risk of developing Parkinson's disease.[1] It may actually be one of the earliest symptoms. The cause of depression in PD remains poorly understood. It may be a primary type of depression that is intrinsic to the disease and accompanying changes in brain chemistry. Or alternatively it is a secondary or reactive depression to the discovery that one has a chronic progressive disease. In addition, the effect of PD medications is not well understood. Some individuals may notice a worsening of depression as their PD treatment begins, while others may have an improvement. Close monitoring by you and your family, friends, colleagues, and health-care providers can be helpful in determining if there are significant changes and if they need to be treated. (See Day 5 for more information on depression and PD.)

Dopamine is the **neurotransmitter** that gets all of the attention, but several other important brain chemicals are also affected by PD. **Serotonin, norepinephrine,** and **acetylcholine** all have an impact on our mental state.

Your doctor or psychiatrist may suggest medication as a way to deal with the chemical imbalance that PD is creating in your brain. One group of anti-depressant medications, called **selective serotonin reuptake inhibitors (SSRIs)**—which includes Prozac and Zoloft—has helped many people with Parkinson's enjoy much happier, more fulfilling lives.

Another neurochemical that may be altered in PD is acetylcholine, which is important for memory. In the advanced stages of PD, there may be loss of acetylcholine in the brain and the presence of significant memory problems severe enough to be called **dementia**. I think that this is one of the biggest fears of all people with Parkinson's and of our families. Research is ongoing to determine factors related to dementia in PD and the utility in PD of memory-enhancing medications currently used to treat Alzheimer's patients.

If you are experiencing feelings of anxiety, loss of motivation or focus, difficulty remembering things, irritability, or other behaviors that are not typically part of your personality, be sure to let your health-care provider know as soon as possible so you can begin to explore treatment options.

Gastrointestinal problems

PD can affect your entire **gastrointestinal tract (GI)** from top to bottom, so to speak. Rigid muscles in your throat and esophagus can make you choke and possibly aspirate food (inhale into your lungs). Your stomach may empty slower than it did before PD, which can cause bloating and nausea. If your upper GI tract is slow, chances are good that the lower portion will be as well, making constipation a problem. You can help to ensure that your bowel movements are regular by drinking plenty of water, getting enough fiber in your diet, and exercising routinely.

Loss of facial expression

When your facial muscles become rigid, your ability to express your feelings without speaking is impaired or lost altogether. This loss of expression is called **facial masking.**

We don't often realize how much we have come to rely on visual cues to determine another person's feelings. I had not thought too much about it until I was at a leadership-training seminar a few years ago. We were all required to give presentations and receive feedback from the group about how persuasive we were. I gave my spiel on PD and mentioned masking as one of the features of the disease. The trainer thanked me for telling him, because had he not known, he would have concluded that I was not very interested in my topic. Now whenever I do any public speaking about PD, I make a point of explaining this common feature of PD.

Masking has affected my relationship with my husband. When I am angry, I tend to set my jaw in a stony expression. (I am working to overcome this behavior.) Unfortunately, PD can cause this same look. It has taken my husband a long time to adjust to this, but now if I appear to be scowling, he will ask me if I'm angry. In most cases, I am not. This is one of the subtle, frustrating ways that PD can affect all of your relationships.

Some people with Parkinson's also develop what I call the "deer-in-the-headlights" look—a blank stare that seems to go with masked facial features.

Loss of sense of smell

No one knows the reason for this, but many people with Parkinson's (as many as 70 to 90 percent) report that they have little or no sense of smell.[2] This phenomenon is also common in Alzheimer's disease patients.

The relative significance of this finding remains to be seen. In January 2005, the University of Pennsylvania began recruiting participants for a study, "Olfactory Function in Relatives of Patients with Parkinson's Disease."[3] This research trial will send a "scratch-and-sniff" smell test to willing parents or siblings of people with PD, with the goal of finding a cost-effective screening tool to identify people at risk for PD.

Dale's experience

DALE WAS in his early thirties and working as a call-center manager for a large telecommunications firm when he noticed that he seemed to be losing his sense of smell. He saw a doctor, who performed some tests and gave him a clean bill of health. About two years later, he began experiencing pain and rigidity in his shoulder. In April 1994, more than four years after noting the changes in his ability to detect odors, he was diagnosed with PD.

Soft voice/slurred speech/choking

You may notice that people ask you to repeat things or to speak louder. PD can affect the depth of breathing and therefore the force of air to generate normal speech. The throat muscles used for speech may not work as well together as they did in the past either, so your speech may be slurred at times. I've learned that if I feel as if I am yelling, I am probably speaking just loudly enough to be heard properly. I also need to pronounce words carefully, particularly when I am tired. According to the National Parkinson Foundation, the majority (60 to 90 percent) of PD patients will experience some effects on their speech during the course of their disease, and at least half will have trouble swallowing. Loss of coordination of your swallowing muscles can also cause choking while you are eating or drinking.

In hindsight, I realize that choking was one of my early symptoms. At the time, I chalked it up to being a young mother accustomed to having to eat quickly. In fact, I had a very embarrassing situation before being diagnosed. My "team" of six coworkers was having lunch with our new executive director at a nearby Vietnamese restaurant run by the family of one of the team. While munching on an egg roll, I suddenly began to choke. My new boss performed the **Heimlich maneuver** on the spot and literally saved my life. Talk about a way to make an impression!

Small, cramped handwriting

Some people will notice that their handwriting has gotten smaller (**micrographia**) before they are diagnosed. Many others will look back after they have been told they have PD and see that a distinct change in their handwriting had occurred long before they received a diagnosis. A number of historians have hypothesized that Adolf Hitler had Parkinson's disease, based on changes noted in his handwriting over the years. His other symptoms included a tremor that has been noticed in films, and flexed posture of one of his arms.

Changes in walking

You may do "the Parkie shuffle," sliding your feet when you walk, instead of lifting them. You may trip often. Or you may lean forward and take quick but small steps. Doctors call this type of movement **festination**.[4] I had a consistent tightness in my left hamstring that no amount of stretching would help—until I began taking Sinemet. Because of that, I would take a regular stride with my right leg but a shorter step with my left, dragging it the rest of the way to catch up. This still happens when my medication is not working (known as an **off time**) or when I am very tired. I always feel like Marty Feldman's character Igor in the movie *Young Frankenstein*.

IN A SENTENCE:

> *Early symptoms of PD can affect your speech, sense of smell, movement, digestion, and many other body functions.*

learning

PD's Effects on the Brain

AS YOU now know, Parkinson's disease occurs in a part of the brain called the substantia nigra. This part of the brain makes dopamine, which then goes to the **corpus striatum** in another area of the brain. The corpus striatum acts as a sort of central switchboard for messages to our muscles (see figure below). When the dopamine system is not working, our muscles get messages telling them to move more than we really want them to, so we have tremors; or the muscles are told to tense up, causing rigidity. And sometimes they are told to stop moving altogether, resulting in a phenomenon known as "freezing."

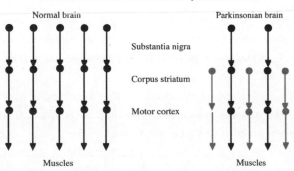

Difference between a normal brain and a parkinsonian brain

Reprinted from Natalie Kontakos and Julie Stokes, "Parkinson's Disease—Recent Developments and New Directions."

The black symbols indicate signals about muscle movement going successfully from the substantia nigra (where dopamine is produced) through relay centers in the corpus striatum and **motor cortex** areas of the brain. The gray symbols represent the loss of dopamine in the signaling process.

"Brain Ballet"—The Dance of the Neurotransmitters

AS THEIR name indicates, neurotransmitters carry messages from the part of the brain in which they are generated to other parts of the body. Like oil for the Tin Man character in *The Wizard of Oz*, dopamine's job is to keep your muscles moving freely and smoothly without conscious thought. You may have noticed that tasks or movements that used to be automatic now require a great deal of thought and concentration.

Here is a less technical way to look at the relationship between dopamine and acetylcholine. I like to think of it as a dance—a ballet—because when it's working, their relationship allows us to move with ease and grace.

Dopamine. Consider this neurotransmitter to be the prima ballerina, or lead dancer, in our brain ballet.

Acetylcholine. This messenger is her consort, her dance partner. Together, they engage in a pas de deux to tell your muscles how to move. Under normal conditions, dopamine and acetylcholine take turns leading, depending on the "dance steps" required. Parkinson's disease disrupts this dance rhythm.

Monoamine oxidase (MAO-B). This enzyme's job is to "cut in" on a regular basis and clear dopamine from the stage.

Most drug treatments act to increase the number of dopamine dance partners available or to prevent acetylcholine from going solo. Some medications, called **MAO inhibitors,** keep MAO enzymes from breaking down the existing supply of dopamine.

If this metaphor doesn't work for you, and/or you want more detailed scientific information, there are numerous resources available in print and online. See the Resources section of this book for a list of good ones.

Attack of the free radicals?

One theory as to the cause of PD is that free radicals damage or kill dopamine-producing neurons. **Free radicals** are produced by normal body chemical reactions and are short one electron, so they go out looking for one to steal. Think of them as "vampire molecules." They are especially fond of metals, such as iron. The process by which free radicals take other cells captive for their electrons is called **oxidation. Antioxidants** are the equivalent of crucifix-brandishing molecules; their job is to quash the free radicals.

Lewy bodies are a pathological hallmark of Parkinson's disease. They are not typically visible with current imaging technology. They can be seen under a microscope when an autopsy is conducted, but at that point it is obviously too late for any treatment. Lewy bodies are clumps of material that contain proteins, such as **alpha-synuclein**. There are several theories as to the possible role alpha-synuclein may play in causing PD. First, it may cause leaks in cell membranes, which could lead to cell death.[5] Second, buildup of the protein could cause what amounts to the clogging of a cell's "garbage disposal" system. Or an overabundance of alpha-synuclein could cause toxic levels in the cell, killing **neurons** that way. To date, alpha-synuclein and Lewy bodies remain part of the smoking gun that researchers are looking for.

IN A SENTENCE:

> *Parkinson's disease disrupts the brain's delicate chemistry and can alter its landscape as well.*

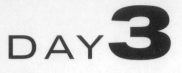

living

To Medicate or Not to Medicate

WHEN YOUR doctor gave you your diagnosis, one of the first questions that popped into your head after "Why me?" and "What caused this to happen?" was probably "How is PD treated?"

Do you have to take medication?

At some point, you will have to start taking medication. However, there is no hard-and-fast rule about when you should begin taking it, because everyone has different symptoms and their disease progresses at different rates. After being diagnosed, many people go for months or years before they start medication of any kind. It's a decision that you and your doctor should make together. Your involvement is important, because only you can decide how much of any symptom you can tolerate, and you will be the one who is going to take the medication and experience any side effects.

First, find a doctor familiar with PD

It's important to find a doctor who is experienced in treating Parkinson's patients. This may be your internist or general practitioner, but in all likelihood you will see a neurologist (a medical doctor who specializes in injuries and illnesses that affect the central nervous system) or a movement disorders specialist (a health-care provider, usually a neurologist, who has been trained to treat diseases that affect the way your body moves, such as multiple sclerosis, and **amyotrophic lateral sclerosis** [also known as ALS or Lou Gehrig's disease]).

PD Treatment Has Come a Long Way

SOMETIMES IT can be easy to get frustrated with medical science and the lack of more effective treatments for PD. The next time you find yourself falling into that trap, consider this: prior to the 1960s, no one knew about dopamine, its role in muscle movements, and the loss of dopamine-producing neurons in the development of Parkinson's disease.[1] That meant that very little could be done for people with PD and the long-term prognosis was poor. These days there are quite a few medications available and many different theories about which to try first and when.

Beliefs differ about what to try and when

Some doctors prescribe medication upon diagnosis (or even as a tool to help diagnose PD; more on that later in the chapter). Others believe that drugs, especially levodopa, should be delayed as long as possible because of their side effects and to possibly extend their period of effectiveness. Since PD affects everyone differently, there is no universal "right" answer. This is one reason that it is critical for you to trust your health-care provider.

An antidepressant may be prescribed first

Because depression is very common in people with Parkinson's (see Day 6), you may start on an **antidepressant**. Such medications will not help symptoms such as tremor or rigidity, but they may help you to sleep and, of course, improve your mood. Getting enough rest and maintaining your spirits can actually reduce your symptoms and thus delay the need for other drugs.

Give medications time to work

With the exception of **apomorphine,** which is is injected into the skin to deal with an episode of freezing in advanced PD, Parkinson's medications do not work instantaneously. (And I can almost guarantee that in your first year of dealing with a PD diagnosis, you will not be taking apomorphine). You may need to take a medication for days or even weeks to determine whether it is beneficial. This waiting is usually difficult and provokes anxiety. Keeping a **drug diary** can help you to deal with those emotions, as well as document the efficacy and side effects of the medication. Even when a medication is working properly, it may not relieve all of your symptoms. There is no "magic bullet" that is guaranteed to make all PD patients feel as if they do not have the disease.

> I didn't want to take any medication. I said that I was OK, could wait, etc. After starting the Amantadine, I could not believe the difference in my life. Why did I fight taking it so long? I was allowing myself to curl up and sleep from all of the fatigue. Now I look at PD as a hurdle in my life, that I just have to learn to overcome some physical difficulties. And I am enjoying my life more than ever before. My life and my family have greater meaning. —ROBERTA, *diagnosed at 44*

Never stop taking a medication without your doctor's approval

Once you have been taking a medication for several weeks, do not abruptly stop taking it without the advice and supervision of your doctor. Doing so can really throw you into a tailspin of symptoms from which it is difficult to recover. Make sure that you always have extra medication on hand for trips and vacations.

Anticholinergic medications

These medications are the oldest in the arsenal of Parkinson's drugs. They block acetylcholine (dopamine's counterpart), which allows dopamine to control your movements.

They are not used much these days, because more effective medicines and ones with fewer side effects are now available. Still, certain people may get some benefit for tremor and other motor problems.

Side effects associated with these medications include dry mouth, blurred vision, constipation, drowsiness, retention of urine, confusion, and **hallucinations.** Because they can cause confusion, these drugs should not be used by elderly people or those already experiencing cognitive problems.[2]

Drugs That Your Doctor May Prescribe

Dopamine Agonists	Dopamine Precursors/ Replacements
Bromocriptine (Parlodel®) Pergolide (Permax®) Pramipexole (Mirapex®) Ropinirole (Requip®)	Levodopa (Larodopa®) Carbidopa-levodopa (Sinemet® or Atamet® generic brand) Extended-release carbidopa-levodopa (Sinemet CR®)
COMT inhibitors Tolcapone (Tasmar®) Entacapone (Comtan®)	**Anticholinergic drugs** Trihexyphenidyl HCL (Artane®) Benztropine mesylate (Cogentin®) Procyclidine (Kemadrin®) Biperiden HCL (Akineton®)
Antiviral (prescribed for dyskinesia) Amantadine (Symmetrol®)	**MAO-B inhibitors** Selegiline (Eldepryl®)

For a more complete list of medications and possible side effects, see Appendix 1. See Day 6 and Day 7 for lists of medications used for depression, anxiety, and dementia.

Just like medications prescribed for other illnesses, the drugs used to treat the symptoms of PD can affect your entire body, not merely the specific area causing your PD. For instance, nearly any medication taken by mouth can irritate your stomach. And since PD drugs are intended to affect your brain chemistry, it should come as no surprise that they can change the way your brain regulates more than they do just movement.

Common side effects of PD medications

HERE'S A list of some of the most common side effects you may run into when taking PD medications:

○ Nausea and/or vomiting
○ Orthostatic hypotension (low blood pressure), which can cause dizziness or fainting if you stand up too quickly from a seated or prone position
○ Depression, anxiety, and apathy. If you already had a history of anxiety, dopamine agonists may make the condition worse
○ Cognitive changes, such as difficulty remembering things, feeling confused, and having trouble with concentration
○ Changes in sleep habits, like insomnia or drowsiness and vivid dreams

Levodopa

L-3,4-dihydroxyphenylalanine, or "L-dopa," is found naturally in plants and animals and is derived from the amino acid tyrosine. In drug form, L-dopa is referred to as "levodopa." Developed in 1967, levodopa is considered the most effective method for treating symptoms of PD because it attempts to provide your body with the dopamine it needs. Other drugs help your body make the most of the dopamine you have, or act on other neurotransmitters to balance your brain chemistry.

Dopamine cannot cross the blood-brain barrier, which is why doctors can't administer it. Instead, levodopa is used. The addition of carbidopa reduces the amount of levodopa needed and keeps it from being converted to dopamine before it reaches the brain. Even so, only 1 to 10 percent of levodopa actually reaches its target area. The amount of carbidopa and levodopa in the medication is expressed as a ratio and should be listed on the label on the prescription bottle. The most common dosages are 25/100 or 25/250; in other words, 25 parts carbidopa per 100 or 250 parts levodopa.

Sinemet is the commercial name for the drug combination of carbidopa to levodopa. Outside of the United States, it is marketed under the name

Madopar. Most everyone takes Sinemet at some point during his or her journey with PD. If Sinemet does not work when first prescribed, that is a sign to your doctor that you may not have Parkinson's disease; you may have another form of parkinsonism or some other disorder altogether.

Drugs for dyskinesia

Antidyskinesia medications are drugs that help to control **dyskinesia,** the involuntary movements that are made worse by levodopa therapy (see the Learning section of Day 3 for more on levodopa therapy).

Amantadine (Symmetrel®) is an antiviral drug that was originally developed to ward off influenza but was found to have properties that alleviate some of the symptoms in the early stages of PD and can help to minimize dyskinesias induced by Sinemet in later stages. No one knows why amantadine improves these symptoms, but I know from personal experience that it can be very beneficial.

Side effects of amantadine include both insomnia and daytime fatigue; edema (swelling/water retention), especially in the feet; retention of urine; as well as effects common to many other PD medications (dizziness, depression, anxiety, and hallucinations). Amantadine can also cause **livedo reticularis,** red or purple blotches or netlike patterns, usually beginning on the legs. These blotches are caused by constriction of blood vessels in the area. The condition goes away if you discontinue the medication, although it may take weeks or months for it to disappear completely.

Drug holidays

ON RARE occasions, your doctor may take you off a medication temporarily to allow side effects to subside. This is called a **drug holiday.** For example, I had been taking Amantadine for my dyskinesia. It was very helpful but I developed livedo reticularis, so Dr. Tuite took me off of it for two months. The condition went away and I began taking Amantadine again at a much lower dose. I cannot emphasize enough how important it is to take your medication as directed, and don't ever stop taking it abruptly. Do not attempt a drug holiday without medical supervision.

COMT inhibitors

The two main COMT inhibitors available are **entacapone (Comtan®)** and **Tolcapone (Tasmar®)**. These medications work by inhibiting (stopping) an enzyme, catechol-O-methyl transferase (COMT), to allow more levodopa to be converted into dopamine. This process can help with "wearing off" effects of Sinemet that occur after years of taking that medication. These drugs are always taken with carbidopa/levodopa, because they have no direct effect on Parkinson's symptoms.

Tasmar is rarely used now because of the risk of liver damage as well as other potential side effects (severe diarrhea, dyskinesia, and hallucinations, to name a few).[3] It is prescribed only to people who cannot tolerate other medications and who do not have a prior history of liver disease. If your doctor prescribes this medication, you will be required to undergo liver-enzyme tests on a regular basis. People over age seventy-five are at increased risk of hallucinations from Tasmar.[4]

MAO-B inhibitors

Monoamine oxidase inhibitors (MAOI or MAOs) block enzymes that break down dopamine in your brain, which allows the dopamine that you have to work longer. MAO-A and MAO-B drugs block different enzymes in different parts of the brain.

Selegiline is an MAO-B inhibitor and historically has been prescribed as Sinemet begins showing signs of wearing off. However, research is now being conducted on the neuroprotective potential of the drug. (See Month 12 for more information.)

Selegiline has many of the same potential side effects as other PD meds: nausea, vomiting, or diarrhea; insomnia or vivid dreams; anxiety; and dry mouth. It should not be taken with Demerol®, a narcotic painkiller, because the combination of the two drugs can cause "stupor, muscle rigidity, severe agitation . . . elevated temperature . . . and death."[5] (This is a very extreme example of why keeping a complete medication list with you at all times is a good idea. Your neurologist would know that you shouldn't take Demerol, but your general practitioner or an emergency-room physician, who might treat you for an injury, would not necessarily know about this risk. Many people with PD see a variety of health-care providers and may have medication prescribed by all of them.)

Dopamine agonists

Although this class of medications has been around since the 1970s,[6] they came into widespread use for PD in the United States only in the late 1990s. **Dopamine agonists (DAs)** are not actually converted into dopamine, as levodopa is. Instead, they mimic dopamine—that is, they are structurally similar to dopamine and so can act on dopamine **receptors** in the brain.

At first, dopamine agonists were used after levodopa therapy alone was no longer effective. Now DAs are often the first medication prescribed for PD, especially for young-onset Parkinson's. Many PD patients do fine for several years on a DA alone; others take Sinemet, often with a DA or other medications.

Despite the ability to simulate dopamine and address many of the symptoms of PD, research thus far suggests that levodopa is still more effective on motor symptoms. Levodopa has more motor-related side effects, but DAs have many cognitive and other impacts. You and your doctor must discuss the options and be willing to modify your plan as needed.

ASLEEP AT THE WHEEL

Sleep attacks, or **sudden onset of sleep (SOS),** are common with dopamine agonists, especially those that are not derived from ergot (pramipexole and ropinirole). Older men who have had PD for a while and have a history of sleep problems have the greatest risk of sleep attacks.[7]

DOPAMINE AGONISTS MAY INDUCE ADDICTIVE OR OBSESSIVE BEHAVIOR

Early research speculated that the pathological behaviors (shopping, gambling, hypersexuality, food cravings) that were seen in some patients who were taking dopamine agonists were rare.[8] Now scientists are acknowledging that these behaviors are not so rare and that more research should be done regarding these effects.[9] If you experience any of these behaviors—or care partners, if you observe any such changes—be sure to tell your doctor so that you can discuss options for dealing with them.

IF DOPAMINE AGONISTS HAVE SO MANY SIDE EFFECTS, WHY TAKE THEM?

Agonists are used to buy time until better treatments or a cure is found. Remember, not everyone will experience all of these side effects. The average length of time people with Parkinson's can take Sinemet without experiencing "on/off" periods or dyskinesia is five years. If you are a young person with PD, you will need to think about whether you want to put off taking Sinemet for a while in exchange for potentially falling asleep at the wheel or becoming a sex maniac. There are ways to avoid falling asleep at the wheel, and additional medications can mitigate obsessive-compulsive urges, but there aren't any viable long-term alternatives to Sinemet at this time. Dopamine agonists are also used to treat **restless legs syndrome,** a nighttime condition in which you feel like your legs need to keep moving. This disorder affects both people who have Parkinson's and those who don't.

Choosing a treatment

There are always philosophical debates about treatment options for any illness. Let's look at a non-PD-related example. Let's say you are forty-something years old and you find yourself holding the newspaper out from your body so that you can read it. Time for bifocals or reading glasses, right? Some people think that giving in and using glasses will hasten their eye muscle "weakness" and result in the need for increasing strength of lenses. They can't see right now, but they are hoping that something will come along later that will save them from wearing glasses. I call this the "I'll do it my way" aggressive approach, also known as "You're not the boss of me." Others think that since everyone else their age wears reading glasses, they should have some, too. They haven't seen an optometrist yet but assume they don't need to, because everyone knows that once you hit forty, your near vision goes. I consider this approach the "Okay, whatever you say, boss" or "herd mentality" method of decision making. I encourage you to consider a third approach to deciding on a treatment plan: "Let's make a deal."

I believe in gathering as much information as you can, getting input from people you trust, and then talking with your care partner and health-care provider about what you feel is best for you. My deal with you as a reader is that I will try to provide the information and the encouragement, and then you need to take it the rest of the way to find the best care and treatment for you.

The Financial "Side Effects" of Medications

Treating PD is not cheap! The National Parkinson Foundation estimates that patients spend an average of $2,500 per year on medications. For most everyone, this is a significant expense. Here are a few suggestions on how to minimize your medication costs:

Ask for samples. When your health-care provider prescribes a new medication, ask her if there are any sample packages of the drug. This can not only minimize your costs; it can reduce the number of partially full prescription bottles in your medicine chest.

Get the generic form of the drug, if there is one.*

Use mail-order service if it is available through your clinic or insurance provider. It is almost always much cheaper to get a three-month supply of a medication, and for drugs like Sinemet, which we know we're going to be taking for a long time, this makes a lot of sense. Do not do this until you have been on the medication for a month or two and know that it works for you and that your body will tolerate it.

Ask some pharmaceutical companies for help. Many of the pharmaceutical companies have programs to assist people who do not have health insurance or who cannot otherwise afford medication. Look under Day 3 in Resources for a list of assistance programs funded by drug manufacturers.

---

* Be aware that there are a few people who are unusually sensitive to dyes, binders, and flavorings in medications. (I happen to be one of them.) For us, just any old brand won't do. I have learned the hard way that there is one generic brand of carbidopa-levodopa that I can take. With other brands, I have to take literally twice as much, and even then the effect is not beneficial. If you notice a sudden change in the efficacy of your medication or develop a rash or other side effects after getting a prescription refilled, talk to the pharmacist. Have her check the formulary (the approved list of medication that a health plan or clinic has in stock and will reimburse). Generally, medications ordered "off-formulary" have to be approved in advance by the insurance company or they will not be covered.

When you're taking more than one medication

You may be wondering what could happen if you are taking two or three medications that all have drowsiness or dizziness as potential side effects. Will that make you two or three times dizzier or drowsier? Possibly. That is why you, or you and your care partner as a team, should keep a drug diary to record your reactions. It's another reason why you should make sure that your doctor and especially your pharmacist are aware of all of the prescription and **over-the-counter (OTC) medications** you are taking. For more information on possible drug interactions, see Week 3.

I wish I had known

Some medications can bring on obsessive-compulsive behaviors. Susan says that Permax brought on her husband's compulsions:

> Gambling was the biggest problem. When I think back, it was sex, then shopping, then doing our basement over like a night club (it's over the top; we have a musical family), then the gambling. Had we known beforehand about possible OCD [obsessive-compulsive disorder], we would have had our guard up. The gambling was totally out of character. It had gone on for a year before we finally mentioned it to the doctor, and he wasn't surprised! Of course since all this, we've read and heard this is pretty common! NO ONE SAID A WORD!!! —SUSAN, *care partner of husband diagnosed at age 41*

Many premenopausal women with PD report that their symptoms worsen or their medication doesn't seem to work as well two or three days before their menstrual period begins and through the first couple days of their period.

Having a cold or the flu can also affect your PD, since your body is under stress. OTC products can interfere with medications, too. (Sometimes there is a warning about this on the package, but not always.)

IN A SENTENCE:

> *Some physicians will start you on drug therapy immediately, while others delay it as long as possible. The jury is still out as to which plan is more effective.*

learning

Things to Expect if You're Taking Sinemet

IF YOU and your doctor have decided that it's time to begin taking Sinemet, there are a few things you should know about the medication (aside from the fact that there is a very good chance that it will help you to start feeling much better very soon!).

Levodopa has increased PD life expectancy

Before levodopa and dopamine agonists appeared on the scene, people with PD had a life expectancy of ten to twenty years after onset, and when they died, it was due to complications from being unable to move (e.g., pneumonia or urinary tract infections).[10] Now our average life expectancy is nearly the same as those who don't have PD.

People with young-onset Parkinson's should work with their health-care provider and weigh the benefits and risks of taking Sinemet and other PD medications for possibly thirty to forty years.

More is not better

When doctors initially began prescribing Sinemet, they gave patients as much as they could tolerate. Now, in order to maximize the term of effectiveness and minimize the side effects, doctors will establish the lowest dose that provides you with relief. The dosage will then be increased slowly, often in combination with other medications, as your disease progresses.

Not all symptoms respond equally

Some PD symptoms respond to Sinemet better than others. Rigidity and bradykinesia can usually be relieved with levodopa. Some people will find that it helps reduce their tremors. Balance problems are the symptom least likely to be improved by Sinemet. Secondary symptoms such as gastrointestinal problems, sexual dysfunction, speech problems, and depression/anxiety are also not improved.[11]

Avoid taking Sinemet on a full stomach

Even though it may cause nausea, Sinemet should not be taken with a meal, especially one with a lot of protein. A full stomach can interfere with the drug's absorption. Be sure to drink a full glass of water. If you find that the medication makes you feel sick, eat a couple of soda crackers just before taking the medication. Most people find that Sinemet is most effective when it is taken forty-five to sixty minutes before a meal or at least two hours after eating.

Levodopa is found in some foods

Although L-dopa occurs naturally in some foods, there is no current proven method of getting enough of the chemical through our diet to control our PD. Fava beans are known to be high in levodopa, and some people with Parkinson's claim to experience a benefit from eating a diet high in fava beans. The levodopa content of fava beans can vary widely based on several factors, such as the amount of rainfall and sunlight the plant receives, the soil type, and where it is grown. Fresh green beans and the pod that surrounds them contain the most levodopa, although some is still present in dried mature beans. You would have to eat about ½ cup of fresh beans or 3 ounces (84 grams) of drained, canned beans to get somewhere between 50 and 100 milligrams of levodopa.[12] Fava beans come with their own risks. Eating the raw beans can induce an allergic reaction in some people. There are also some people who lack an enzyme needed to digest fava beans. This genetic disease, known as **"favism,"** can cause a potentially fatal called hemolytic anemia. If you are interested in adding fava beans to your diet, discuss it with your doctor—particularly if you take any MAO inhibitor medications.

Another legume, Mucuna pruriens, has been used in ancient Indian Ayurvedic medicine as a naturally derived source of levodopa. It is being investigated now by Western medical practitioners as a viable alternative to Sinemet.

How soon is too soon to start taking Sinemet?

Scientific opinion is divided on the subject of when to begin levodopa therapy. The duration of the effect of a dose of Sinemet tends to decline rapidly after about five years of therapy, so many people, particularly those with **young-onset Parkinson's disease (YOPD)**—sometimes called **early-onset Parkinson's disease**, choose to delay their use of Sinemet as long as possible. (When a dose no longer works as long, this phenomenon is called "motor fluctuation.") On the other hand, if your existing treatment regime is not helping your symptoms and your doctor recommends Sinemet, you should at least give it a try. If levodopa therapy does not help your symptoms at all, then you need to let your physician know. It may indicate that you have a form of parkinsonism that is not idiopathic Parkinson's disease.

If Sinemet doesn't work

Since there is no definitive test for PD and many other forms of parkinsonism, your body's response to Sinemet remains the best criterion for establishing a diagnosis. Like the English language, parkinsonism contains nearly as many exceptions as "rules," but in general, people with idiopathic PD will get some relief from their symptoms from Sinemet. If you don't, you may have some other form of parkinsonism.

Other Types of Parkinsonism

HERE IS a brief description of other types of parkinsonism. For more information or additional resources on these other conditions, contact WE MOVE (see their Web site and other contact information in Resources).

FORMS OF PARKINSONISM/ PARKINSON'S SYNDROME

○ Drug-induced parkinsonism
○ Post-encephalitic parkinsonism
○ Manganese poisoning/"welders' disease"

We know the causes of these conditions, and we know that they generally respond to Sinemet. I do not know why there has not been more effort put into naming conventions that would reduce or eliminate confusion for patients and the general public.

PARKINSON'S PLUS (PD+) DISORDERS OR ATYPICAL PARKINSON'S

These conditions have some symptoms in common with PD but have additional health effects that differentiate them.[13] PD+ disorders are rare compared to PD. As stated earlier, they are even more difficult to diagnose than PD, and significant differences are usually not noticed until a person's condition has deteriorated markedly.

Primary differences between idiopathic PD and PD+:

○ Idiopathic PD responds well to Sinemet, and PD+ disorders do not.
○ PD+ tends to progress much more quickly.
○ Lewy bodies are found in the brains of most people believed to have died with PD. Lewy bodies are not found in the brains of people with PD+.
○ Most of the autopsies of PD brains also show significant loss of dopamine-producing neurons in the substantia nigra.

MULTIPLE SYSTEM ATROPHY (MSA)

To put it plainly, this means that several important body systems stop functioning properly. There are three forms: Music legend Johnny Cash suffered from **Shy-Drager syndrome**, which is marked by failure of the autonomic nervous system, which regulates your blood pressure, bladder, temperature, and unconscious or "automatic" systems in the body. Primary symptoms of **striatonigral degeneration** include slowed movements and rigidity. **Olivopontocerebellar atrophy** is characterized by dramatic changes in balance, coordination, and speech.[14] For every hundred people who have PD, five have MSA.[15] As is the case with idiopathic PD, the causes of these various forms of MSA are unknown.

PROGRESSIVE SUPRANUCLEAR PALSY (PSP)

The hallmarks of PSP include early and severe balance problems, with frequent falls; slowed movements; speech and swallowing problems, and inability to make your eyes look downward. There can be personality and cognitive changes, too, such as difficulties with memory and abstract thinking.[16] This condition progresses quickly. The actor/pianist Dudley Moore had PSP.

Men are more likely than women to develop PSP. There are five cases of PSP for every hundred people with PD.[17]

Dosage information

Sinemet is a combination of carbidopa and levodopa. The ratio of the two components is used when describing your dose. For example, when the nurse reviews your medication list at each doctor visit, you might say, "I take one tablet of Sinemet CR [controlled-release] 50/200 when I get up in the morning and one tablet of Sinemet 25/100 around 3:00 p.m."

There are generic versions of the drug available that are much cheaper than the name brand. For the purposes of this book, I will use the term "Sinemet" to refer to both the brand name and the generic, unless stated otherwise.

You may get nauseated when you first begin taking Sinemet. The physician may urge you to "tough it out" for a couple of weeks to see if the effect goes away by itself, or she may prescribe some additional carbidopa in the form of Lodosyn®. If this fails to solve the problem, there are other compounds that may be helpful, such as Tigan®, Zofran®, or Domperidone®.

The dyskinesia dance

If at any point while taking Sinemet or other antiparkinsonian medications you or others notice that your hands, head, or shoulders are writhing or jerking involuntarily, you are experiencing dyskinesia (Greek for "abnormal movement"). These movements are a by-product of the medication and the disease. In my case, I was not the first to notice that I was having dyskinesias. In fact, it was my then-three-year-old son, Bennett, who asked me one day as we were on our way to buy shoes for him at the Mall of America, "Why are you doing that with your head, Mommy?" When I asked what he meant, he nodded and wobbled his head—what I have come to call the "dashboard dog" movement (for those of you who may remember the veloured plastic hounds that used to be sold to adorn your car's dashboard and that lolled their heads with the rhythm of the road). When I mentioned this to my husband, he said, "Oh yeah, I've noticed that. For a while now, your left hand has been moving around like it has a mind of its own."

Keep the following in mind:

○ Not everyone with PD experiences dyskinesia, and not all who are dyskinetic are severely impaired by it.

○ Dyskinesias become increasing more frequent as time goes by, with most developing the movements after eight to ten years of symptoms. It appears that those with young-onset Parkinson's develop dyskinesia and fluctuations in mobility earlier than those with later onset PD. The reason for this remains poorly understood. Fifty-five percent of young-onset Parkinson's patients develop dyskinesia within their first year of levodopa therapy. By the third year of Sinemet use, 74 percent have dyskinesia. In contrast, 28 to 50 percent of older patients (fifty years of age or higher) develop dyskinesia within the first three to five years of levodopa therapy.[18]

When my dyskinesia is particularly bad, as it is while trying to type this passage, it makes completion of my motor task all the more challenging. At first glance, people may wonder if I am doing some strange sort of interpretative dance. My head and arms flail as if I am a marionette being operated by a novice puppetmaster.

Dyskinesia can be embarrassing and painful. It can also burn a lot of calories (and I do not mean that as a benefit). It can turn you into a recluse if you allow it to do so. My view is that if I let my dyskinesia run my life, then the disease wins.

Sometimes the addition of other drugs, such as Amantadine, will reduce dyskinesia. Taking less Sinemet more often can also help. For instance, I now take half of one Sinemet 25/100 about every 90 minutes during the day. This dose regimen has decreased my dyskinesia considerably.

The wearing-off phenomenon

The other phenomenon that occurs over time with Sinemet is that it becomes more difficult to keep an effective amount in the brain at any one time. This is called the **wearing-off phenomenon.** The peaks and valleys result in dyskinesia, which usually occurs when there is a lot of dopamine circulating, and in "off" times, when there is not enough. We usually refer to those times when there is enough dopamine that we can move as "on" times. So if you hear Parkies talking about "on" and "off," we are not talking about light switches!

IN A SENTENCE:

> *Sinemet, the prescription drug that your body converts to its missing dopamine, can bring great relief, but some side effects, too.*

WANTED!

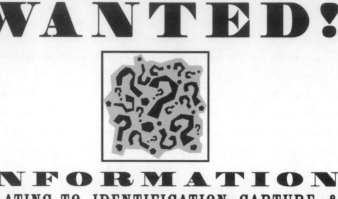

INFORMATION
RELATING TO IDENTIFICATION, CAPTURE, &
ERADICATION
OF THE CAUSE OF
PARKINSON'S DISEASE.

CRIMES: Accessory to murder; torture; theft of mobility, livelihood, hopes, dreams, identity, dignity, financial resources, property, etc.; physical and mental cruelty; hostile takeover of mind and body; kidnapping; trespassing; and other offenses too numerous to list.

VICTIMS: More than one million Americans currently being held hostage.

SUSPECT DESCRIPTION: May be mutant genes (possible aliases may include "parkin," "dardarin"); probable suspects include aluminum, iron, lead, manganese and/or toxic chemicals (members of the "Pesticide Gang"—paraquat, rotenone, maneb—are under investigation or have been indicted for their role in other diseases; chlorinated solvents; and polychlorinated biphenyls, aka PCBs). Suspects may be working together.

REWARD: Eternal gratitude from millions of people who have Parkinson's disease or who care for someone who has it. Billions of dollars saved by American taxpayers. Thousands of people returned to the workforce.

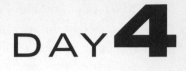

living

Is There PD in Your Family Tree?

INFORMATION ABOUT the role of genetics in PD is rapidly changing and very complicated. I am not a geneticist, and I suspect that neither are most of you. Because of my lack of expertise in this area and the absence of consistent information, this will be a short chapter!

Fifteen to 20 percent of people with Parkinson's have a close relative who has PD or has experienced essential tremor (ET) or some other Parkinson-like symptom.[1] Some researchers include relatives with restless legs syndrome (RLS) as a PD-like symptom.

> Having watched my father in the advanced stages of PD last year, I was able to separate his condition to mine, and in my mind they were separate conditions; his was onset at 62, mine at 44. This has helped me from worrying that I may be like that one day. My attitude: PD will not kill me, something else will. —KARYN, *diagnosed at 44. Her father was diagnosed at 62.*

Many scientists believe that genetic factors are more likely to play a role in "young-onset" or "early-onset" cases of PD, because studies have found that younger patients are more likely to have an affected relative than people diagnosed after age fifty.

Thus far, five genes have been linked to at least some cases of PD: alpha-synuclein, parkin, dardarin, ubiquitin carboxy-terminal hydrolase L1 (UCHL1), and DJ-1.[2]

The genetics of PD are proving to be as variable as the symptoms. Some of the genes implicated in Parkinson's are thought to be dominant, others, recessive.

Dominant traits

With a dominant condition, such as PD caused by the recently discovered gene **dardarin** (also known as LRRK2 or leucine-rich repeat kinase), only one of the two genes that a person has is abnormal. However, it only takes one gene to produce the condition. Two January 2005 studies found that around one in sixty Parkinson's patients have a mutation in gene LRRK2. Researchers believe that this defect is probably responsible for PD in those people, who account for approximately 5 percent of Parkinson's cases with a family history of the disease and another 1.5 to 2 percent of patients with no family history of PD.[3]

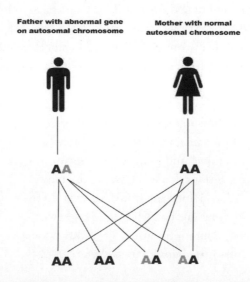

Each pregnancy bears a 50-50 chance of carrying the abnormal gene.

In recessive inherited parkinsonism, both genes need to be abnormal in order to cause full-blown disease. If a person has only one abnormal gene, he would not develop the condition or would only have a mild case.

Genetic researchers had thought that **parkin,** a gene believed to be responsible for at least some cases of young-onset PD, was recessive. However, a recent study looked at nineteen families with late-onset PD in the parent generation and young-onset PD in their children's generation, and twenty-eight individuals with young-onset PD who had no family history of PD.[4] Instead of finding parkin in sixteen of the people with young-onset PD's offspring as expected, they found only one. In contrast, 21 percent of those with young-onset PD had the parkin gene. Now you see what I mean when I said it was complicated.

In the early 1990s, researchers at the Parkinson's Institute in Sunnyvale, California, examined data from a National Academy of Sciences registry of all living twin pairs who had served in World War II. The study was designed to determine whether the rates of PD in identical and fraternal twins were different.

> The results of this study were clear-cut and highly significant. In the twin pairs in whom the disease began after 50 years of age (which constitutes > 95% of all Parkinson's disease), the concordance rates were virtually identical, suggesting that nongenetic factors play an important role in the disease. Interestingly, in patients younger than 50, concordance was dramatically different between monozygotic twins (where four of four twin pairs were concordant) and dizygotic twins (where only 2 of 12 twin pairs were concordant). This strong evidence of heritability in younger-onset patients may well reflect that most of the genetic forms described to date typically have a young onset. The caveat for this component of the study is that the number of twin pairs younger than 50 was small. Overall, the conclusion that can be drawn from the study is that nongenetic factors must play a substantial role in patients with typical Parkinson's disease. Importantly, this study has recently been replicated using the Swedish Twins Registry.[5]

In the families where there are several cases of PD, researchers are attempting to determine whether it may be due to shared environmental exposure (such as well water) or solely due to inheritance of genes. In one large Italian American family it is predicted, based on existing patterns, that half of the children of any family member will develop Parkinson's.[6] This situation suggests a genetic cause. The Mayo clinics in Rochester, Minnesota, and Jacksonville, Florida, have been studying a family in Iowa (referred to as the "Iowa kindred") that has had numerous cases of PD over several generations. In 2004, Mayo researchers identified a genetic defect that they believe is the cause of this family's PD.[7] When a family lives in the same area for generations, other influences, as well as potential causes of genetic mutations, must be considered.

Scientists now know that at least one of these genes affects the production of the protein called alpha-synuclein. Everyone has some synuclein—about 2 percent of all the protein in a normal brain—but obviously, not everyone gets PD. In fact, the lifetime risk of getting PD is also about 2 percent.[8]

In the Parkie brain, alpha-synuclein can build up to form Lewy bodies, which are considered to be a hallmark of Parkinson's disease versus the Parkinson's Plus condition.[9]

What are the odds of genetic transmission?

At this time, most researchers predict only a slightly increased risk for children of people with Parkinson's disease. In her book, *What Your Doctor May Not Tell You About Parkinson's Disease*, Dr. Jill Marjama-Lyons makes these estimates of the risk of developing PD: If there have been no cases of PD in your family, your risk is 1 to 2 percent—the same as everyone else in the United States. If you have a sibling with PD, your chances rise to 5 to 6 percent. If one of your parents has PD, you have a 10 percent chance of getting PD. If you have a parent and a sibling with the disease, your risk is somewhere between 20 and 40 percent.[10] One of the best ways to ensure that we all get better information about PD and genetics is to participate in research trials. (See Month 11 to learn more about participating in research.)

Whether or not PD has a genetic component, the families that experience multiple cases of the disease endure an unspeakable amount of anguish, grief, and pain.

> April 22, 2005
>
> I sit in the quiet of the hospice room, my mother dying of the disease that is also robbing me of my independence, clarity of thought, and physical abilities. To see her struggle with every breath, muscles paralyzed while her limbs shake uncontrollably, seems too cruel a way to die.
>
> I look into the very first set of eyes that met me as I entered this world. The very eyes that have never made me feel a failure or shame but have only encouraged me and loved me. The very same eyes that have seen both her sons laid to rest.
>
> I am planning to donate her brain to the study of Parkinson's disease. To discuss the details at this time seems cruel and morbid. Yet we both would stop at nothing to find the cure to this insidious curse. I touch her head and hope that science appreciates the gift that she is giving them.
>
> My blessing is she has never known of my diagnosis. I could spare her that.
>
> —LINDA COOPER, *diagnosed at age 46. Her mother passed away the next morning.*

Pros and cons of genetic testing

Considerable research, precaution, and compassion will be required in developing an ethical protocol for publicly available genetic testing for PD. There are a host of issues that will need to be resolved, including: what will be done with the genetic information that is collected? Who will have access? For example, will insurance companies be allowed to use the data to exclude someone who has a genetic defect or who is a child of someone with a genetic form of PD? Are there any treatment options available for those who have a gene defect but who are not yet ill? Will counselors be trained and available to help those who test positive to cope with their and their family's future? These are very controversial moral and ethical dilemmas, and they will not be solved easily.

IN A SENTENCE:

> *Some families do have a history of Parkinson's disease, but the condition is not necessarily genetic.*

Environmental Links to PD

I GREW up in small town of less than four thousand people in southwestern Minnesota. I didn't live on a farm, but Jackson is a farming community. Farms in that part of the country tend to grow either corn or soybeans. Conventionally grown soybean and corn are very chemical intensive, using large amounts of fertilizers and herbicides.

At that time, in the late 1970s and early '80s, the primary way for teenagers to earn spending money in the summers was doing fieldwork. Thus, I spent many of my teenage summers detasseling corn or working in soybean fields.

I remember that in my early teens when I first started doing fieldwork, farmers were still "walking beans." This meant that large groups of children and teenagers would get dropped off at one end of the field, and they would walk down the rows to the other side of the field, pulling out or hoeing out as many of the weeds as possible along the way.

By my late teen years, the majority of the farmers had moved on in technology to what was called "spraying beans." This involved a contraption called a "bean buggy"—three to four seats in a row attached to the front of the tractor; each seat had a hose with a long nozzle and trigger. This spray gun was connected to a tank at the back of the tractor. That tank was generally full of an herbicide (usually glyphosate, more commonly known as Roundup®). Many farmers also added a purple dye so that they could see what had been hit. The task at hand was to squirt as many weeds as possible as the tractor progressed along the rows without hitting the soybean plants. It takes a lot less herbicide to kill a bean plant than it does to kill a weed.

I now know that there are explicit instructions on **pesticide** container labels, and I am not attempting to categorize all farmers by saying this, but farmers for whom I worked generally didn't seem to follow the labeled directions all that closely. For instance, we should not have sprayed on windy days, because it would cause the pesticide to drift away from its target and land on other farmers' crops or gardens. Since it is almost always windy in southwestern Minnesota, that instruction was frequently ignored. Also, I recall seeing one farmer using his arm to mix the purple dye into the herbicide in the tank. He died of liver cancer a year or two after that.

Riding on the bean buggy, it was impossible to avoid pesticide exposure. In those days, no one wore any protective gear. We would begin each morning at 5:30 or 6:00 AM, when the fields were still damp and cold from the dew. We would be wearing long pants and jackets or long-sleeved shirts and gloves. But by around 8:30 on a June or July morning, it got to be very hot, and I would be stripped down to my bathing suit and a baseball cap. I would work like that until 1:30 or 2:00 in the afternoon. After that, we would quit because it was too hot. The spraying season lasted two to four weeks, and I would work for several farmers during that time.

I had a great tan those summers, and I had no idea nor gave any thought whatsoever to what I might be exposing myself to, or what the effects might be. After the first day or two of spraying, I could no longer smell the odor of the herbicide. I do remember that when I would come home, my mother would immediately tell me to take a shower because I smelled like chemicals.

I cannot prove that this exposure had anything to do with my onset of Parkinson's disease. I do know that in the years since my fieldwork, I have become much more sensitized to pesticides. I get a headache and easily become nauseated from walking near lawns that have been treated with pesticides.

In addition to the chemical exposure that I had doing fieldwork, I had a major exposure in 1988. I believe that this incident was probably the tipping point in the development of my Parkinson's disease.

In 1988 I was living in Minneapolis and working as the assistant director of a field canvass office (in other words, managing a door-to-door public education and fund-raising effort) for a well-known environmental group. I was very much in love and had just gotten engaged to the man who is now my husband. When I was offered an opportunity to participate in a riverboat tour down the Mississippi with this environmental organization, I jumped at the chance. The purpose of the trip was to educate people along the river about the hazards of the pollution that households and industries were dumping into the river and to talk about ways to minimize or eliminate the pollution.

I participated in the St. Louis, Missouri, to Memphis, Tennessee, leg of the tour. I was working with five or six other people as part of a land-based team that traveled with the boat. Our job was to go out and speak to schoolchildren and community groups about the health and environmental hazards of the toxic chemicals that were going into the river and what they and the local industries could do to reduce it. In addition, we gave tours of the boat at each location and participated in nonviolent direct actions to call attention to the damage that was being caused to the river. We did three direct actions in St. Louis. I participated in two of the three.

One of these actions involved inserting a plug into the discharge pipe from the wastewater sewage treatment plant to symbolically demonstrate that its poisonous flow into the Mississippi River could be stopped.

Six of us took part in that action: four men and two women. The men were in charge of putting the wooden plug (made from several pieces of plywood that were screwed together) in place with hydraulic jacks. The other woman (I'll call her Alice) and I were there as window-dressing. We were to stand on the riverbank holding a banner.

All six of us had been outfitted with dry suits and gloves, but there were only five pairs of rubber boots. I had drawn the short straw, so to speak. Instead of rubber boots, I wore canvas sneakers. Since I didn't expect to be going in the water, it didn't seem like a big deal.

The action went off without a hitch. As the plug was being put into place, security guards from the wastewater treatment plant came down to see what we were doing. They expressed horror that the color of the wastewater, which looked like Mountain Dew, and the smell, which was chemical in nature, were certainly not what one would have expected from a sewage facility. Given instructions not to arrest us, they let us go on with our business. The plug was put in place. Photographs and video footage were shot.

Everyone was in a hurry to return to the boat to get the news out to the media. The photographers were particularly anxious to get back to the boat, so they went in the first inflatable boat. Alice and I remained to wait for the second boat.

During that time, pressure had built up behind the plug. It blew out into the river, and we knew it would be very counterproductive to our message about keeping the river clean if we left it there. My colleague and I waded into the river to retrieve it. Of course, my sneakers filled with toxic water instantly. I waded into the water up to my knees to bring the plug back to the bank and waited for the boat

By the time we had returned to the boat, less than an hour after the exposure to the wastewater, I was feeling like I had the flu. I had a headache and felt achy, nauseous, and very tired. Those symptoms lasted for approximately one week. I know now that those symptoms are indicative of acute pesticide exposure.

I have no way of proving that this exposure caused my Parkinson's disease, but I'm quite certain that it didn't do me any good. I had not really thought about what I might be risking during the action. At twenty-five we tend to think that we are invincible. I was feeling very righteous about my cause and still do. I know that the people who lived downriver from St. Louis and got their drinking water from the river were not given information about what it might contain or a choice about drinking it.

Every day we learn new information about the hazards of the chemicals that we are putting into the environment and into our bodies. I think it's time now to take a step back and reevaluate the process by which we allow chemicals to be introduced into the environment.

Under the current regulatory process in the United States, chemicals are assumed innocent until proven guilty, as if they were human beings on trial for a crime. The onus to prove harm is on us, the public, and we can attempt to prove harm only after it is already been done. This does not seem right to me. I have spent most of the past twenty years trying to change this process.

What pesticides may contribute to PD?

Pesticides may not be the only cause of Parkinson's disease, and not all pesticides may cause Parkinson's disease. However, we do know there are several pesticides—**rotenone, paraquat, maneb**—that do affect

dopamine-producing neurons in laboratory animals. It seems uncon-
scionable that these chemicals are still used and discharged into the environment, our food and our bodies, when we know about this danger and we
know that alternatives are available (also see table on page 55).

Nongenetic risk factors for PD

Most neurologists tell their patients, "genetics loads the gun, but the environment pulls the trigger." Many of us who do not have a family history of
PD or other neurological diseases suspect that a compound or an experience
in our past played a role in the development of our disease. One thing is
clear: you have done nothing intentionally to cause your Parkinson's.

Several life experiences or demographics seem to increase the likelihood
that a person will develop PD. These nongenetic risk factors include:

- Age
- Living in a rural area
- Viral infections
- Working as a welder
- Estrogen deficiency
- Drinking well water
- A serious head injury
- Pesticide exposure
- Working as a farmer

Sources: Marjama-Lyons and Shomon; NIEHS.

PRIOR ILLNESSES

Some cases of PD appear to be caused by viruses. For example, after
World War I, **encephalitis lethargica,** or **sleeping sickness,** swept the
globe. At least 15 million people were infected, and about 6 million developed PD.[11] You may be familiar with the book *Awakenings*, by Dr. Oliver
Sacks, and the subsequent film about his work treating some of the sur-
vivors. This condition, now referred to as **post-encephalitic Parkinson's
disease,** affects the substantia nigra like idiopathic PD, but does not produce Lewy bodies.

Another way in which disease-causing germs might play a role in PD is
by causing **inflammation** in the brain. High fever can be one such source

of inflammation, and many of us had childhood illnesses that included elevated temperatures. There is some speculation that the timing of the inflammation, the fact that it occurred in childhood when our brains and immune systems are not yet fully developed, could have affected the behavior of our dopaminergic neurons later in life.[12]

PHYSICAL INJURY

Head trauma is believed to play a role in at least some cases of parkinsonism, but only in cases of severe injury, usually involving loss of consciousness and a stay in the hospital. Also, the repeated blows to the head received by boxers can induce symptoms of parkinsonism, multiple sclerosis, and Alzheimer's.[13] Muhammad Ali, the world-famous boxer, suffers from parkinsonism but does not have the confusion and other cognitive impairments that are common in boxers who have experienced severe brain injuries.

TOXIC CHEMICALS

We live in a world surrounded by chemicals, so it should surprise no one that some of these substances are suspected of causing Parkinson's disease. Unfortunately, because there are more than eighty thousand chemicals in commerce today, evaluating them one by one will not bring us answers anytime soon.

The first chemical connected with Parkinson's disease was MPTP. In 1982 some San Francisco Bay Area drug users who were attempting to synthesize heroin produced MPTP. Seven of these individuals developed Parkinson-like symptoms within weeks of their exposure to this compound.[14] Today, MPTP is used in the laboratory setting to induce PD-like symptoms in research animals. It is also the standard against which other chemicals suspected of causing PD are measured.

PESTICIDES

As noted earlier, given the widespread use of pesticide products on everything from food crops and lawns to pets and airplanes, each and every one of us is exposed to a variety of these chemicals every day. This chemical soup around us makes it difficult and perhaps somewhat pointless to study one chemical at a time for its potential to cause PD.

Despite the difficulty isolating individual pesticide "bad actors," some specific pesticide products have been strongly linked to PD based on animal research and case studies of people.

Substances in Our Environment Linked to Parkinsons Disease

Chemicals	Heavy Metals
Carbon monoxide	Aluminum
Carbon Disulfide	Copper
Pesticides: Atrazine, Chlorpyrifos	Iron
(e.g., Dursban®), Dieldrin,	Lead
Glyphosate (e.g., Roundup®),	Manganese
Lindane, Mancozeb, Maneb,	Mercury
Paraquat Rotenone	
Polychlorinated biphenyls (PCBs)	
Solvents	
Other	
Endotoxin	

Sources: "Parkinson's Disease and Exposure to Infectious Agents and Pesticides and the Occurrence of Brain Injuries: Role of Neuroinflammation." Bin Liu, Hui-Ming Gao, and Jau-Shyong Hong, Environmental Health Perspectives 111, no 8 (June 2003); "Association of Pesticide Exposure With Neurologic Dysfunction and Disease," Freya Kamel and Jane A. Hoppen, Environmental Health Perspectives 112, no. 9 (June 2004).

CHLORINATED COMPOUNDS ARE FREQUENT SUSPECTS

Many of the chemicals listed here contain chlorine. If free-radical molecules can be likened to vampires because they steal electrons from molecules, chlorine molecules are like demons that take possession of a compound and don't let go. Chlorine does not exist alone in nature, so when chlorine is used as an ingredient or in an intermediate of manufacturing, it is quick to find another element or compound that it can possess. When chlorine bonds with an organic (carbon-based) compound, the result is an organochlorine. Organochlorine compounds are very stable. Humans and animals have a very difficult time "exorcising" or degrading chlorinated compounds, so they get stored in fat and accumulate over time. This process is called **bioaccumulation.**

A database compiled by the **Collaborative on Health and the Environment** suggests that many of the same organochlorines with suspected links to PD have also been implicated as potential causes or contributors to other harmful effects on the brain. These include learning disabilities (polychlorinated biphenyls, or PCBs), brain cancer (lindane), and psychiatric disturbances (**trichloroethylene [TCE],** an organic solvent). Information on how to access this database can be found in the Collaborative on Health and the Environment listing in Resources.

HEAVY HITTERS

Heavy metals are elements—the most basic form that molecules of the same kind can take. (You may remember the periodic table of the elements from your days in high school chemistry.) Elements cannot be broken down any further, but we humans can—and do—redistribute the metals around the planet.

Several heavy metals have been identified as having the potential to cause Parkinson's disease or increase the risk of developing it. All of these metals are associated with other health impacts, especially neurological problems. Those include aluminum, copper, iron, lead, manganese, and mercury.

Some chemicals seem to be directly toxic to neurons. Others may create inflammation in the brain, which reduces the body's resistance to toxins. Another theory is that toxins affect gene expression, meaning that the chemical changes the instructions that the gene gives a particular cell about cell processes, such as cell death.[15]

Ways in which environmental factors can affect the brain

There are many ways in which substances in our environment or events that we experience can affect our brain and lead to PD.

- They create free radicals that destroy neurons or affect the body's system of dealing with free radicals.
- They affect **mitochondria,** which are like the battery or power center in a cell.
- They kill neurons outright.
- They cause the production of alpha-synuclein, the protein that can build up to form Lewy bodies.
- They create inflammation that makes dopamine-producing neurons vulnerable to other "insults."

○ They affect cell receptors, which act as locks or gateways. The job of a receptor may be to open at a particular time to allow an enzyme or neurotransmitter to enter the cell and trigger a series of chemical reactions. Or it may be responsible for keeping out other brain chemicals. Any disruption in this gate-keeping process could have dire consequences, such as blocking instructions telling neurons to produce more dopamine.

How may one be exposed to any of these "Triggers?"

Food, groundwater, and surface water may all contain pesticide residues. Some parts of the country have high levels of heavy metals that are naturally occurring in their water supply. Fertilizer products that contain hazardous industrial waste are another potential source of heavy metals in the environment.

The **National Institute of Neurological Diseases and Sciences (NINDS)** at the National Institutes of Health in Bethesda, Maryland, has undertaken a research study that evaluates pesticide exposure of farmers in three highly agricultural California counties. The **National Agricultural Health Study,** an ongoing project of the National Cancer Institute, the **National Institute of Environmental Health Sciences (NIEHS),** and the U.S. Environmental Protection Agency, has been monitoring the health of nearly ninety-thousand Iowa and North Carolina private pesticide applicators (farmers) and their spouses as well as private pesticide applicators since 1994. Originally the study was meant to cover cancer trends, but now the Parkinson's Institute is doing a study to look at PD trends in these families.

Childhood experiences may be important

Scientists are learning that with many neurological diseases or conditions, what happens to us when we are children—or sometimes even while we are still in our mother's womb—sets the stage for our health outcomes as adults. PD may be no exception. Before adulthood, the organ systems in our bodies are not fully formed or developed. An exposure or event, typically referred to in research as an "insult," may occur and change everything.

Many of us experienced childhood illnesses that were accompanied by high fevers. If the fever caused inflammation of the brain and occurred during a critical phase of our immune system's or our brain's development, our neurons could be permanently affected. It is also possible that such a fever might alter our brain's response to inflammation. Tracking our exposure to viruses is difficult; people may not recall what childhood illnesses they experienced or may not have even been aware that they were sick, especially if the illness occurred when they were young.

Scientists often use the phrase, "The dose makes the poison." Many people—physicians and scientists as well as plain folks like you and me—assume that phrase refers only to the amount of a substance. But if you look at your prescription bottle or read the product insert on an OTC medication, you will see that timing is part of the dosing information.

The timing of risk factors is critical, because our bodies respond differently during various stages of development. Exposure to lead is one example: lead exposure can cause permanent brain damage in children in very small amounts. Why? In part, because their bodies have not fully developed the ability to metabolize lead. Some birth defects have been linked to chemical exposure on a certain day during pregnancy. That same exposure on any other day in the stages of fetal development would not cause those effects. So it is possible that an insult occurring at a time when our brains are being told how many dopaminergic neurons should be formed could change the instructions so that we end up with far fewer than we need to get us through life. Or cells could be programmed to self-destruct, à la *Mission Impossible*.

Many of the chemicals linked to PD are very persistent, meaning our bodies cannot break them down into smaller pieces and get rid of them easily. We may be exposed to some pesticides on a daily basis, although in very small amounts. However, if we can't get rid of them, over time they build up (bioaccumulate) in our bodies. If we reach a certain threshold amount at a particular stage of development, this could trigger PD in us, even as others around us do not develop the disease.

There is still a great deal to be learned about the ways that our genes and the world around us interact. We are all part of one big experiment.

IN A SENTENCE:

> *A number of environmental factors, from pesticides to viruses or injuries, have been linked to the onset of PD.*

Physical Effects of PD

In my next life . . .
Dear Deity,

Does Heaven have a Better Business Bureau?
Does the Universe have a "lemon law"?

I am contacting you to report a defective product.
I would like to speak with someone in your Complaint
    Department about the
physical body issued to me for re-entry to Earth.
This unit is seriously flawed.

It requires far too much maintenance for a 40-year-old
    model.
There are short circuits in the wiring, alternately
causing the chassis to shake, or the wheels to lock up.
Despite the use of high-octane fuel, there have been
frequent fuel intake and exhaust system problems.
Sometimes it has no sense of direction, and
the turn signals don't always work.
Plus it could use a paint job.

I must have some karmic debt in arrears, and
You seem to charge a very high interest rate.
Please advise me of your preferred payment schedule, and
I will budget accordingly with limbs and internal organs.
I want to have that debt paid in full so that maybe next
    time around,
I can have a new, deluxe model with the extended warranty.

©Jackie Hunt Christensen 2004

Common PD symptoms

As with all Parkinson's symptoms, not everyone will experience all of these effects. Some may experience them in mild form; for others, they will be more severe. Once a symptom starts, it may continue for the duration of your disease, but then again, it may not. If you experience one of these symptoms, tell your care partner and health practitioner so you can discuss what to do.

CONSTIPATION AND INCONTINENCE/BLADDER PROBLEMS

PD affects both divisions of the autonomic nervous system (the **sympathetic** and **parasympathetic nervous systems**). Among its many roles, the autonomic system is in charge of smooth muscles, which include the bladder and bowels. This may result in constipation or, in extreme cases, bowel impaction. So this is just one more reason that it is critical that you get enough exercise and drink plenty of water.

DROOLING/EXCESS SALIVA

About 70 percent of PD patients will experience drooling or have excess saliva at some point.[1] This can obviously be embarrassing, but it has no connection to dementia. It can also interfere with your speech and with eating.

To cope with too much saliva, you can try chewing gum or sucking on hard candies. When eating, chew your food slowly and swallow often. (Note: You may also have dry mouth, or too little saliva, which can be caused by medications.)

DYSTONIA

"Dys" means abnormal or irregular; "tonia" refers to muscle tone or tension. With dystonia, your muscles have too much "tone." In other words, they remain tightened or rigid when they should be relaxed. This results in writhing movements and contorted postures. Dystonia is actually a form of dyskinesia.[2] It can affect various parts of your body and cause a great deal of pain. Neck, shoulders, and feet are very common locations for dystonia. There are medications, such as Baclofen®, which may be helpful. Botulinum (**botox**) injections have also been helpful to many people, though some people experience no benefit at all. For those who do benefit from botox injections, the effects can last for weeks or even months.

FATIGUE

You may find yourself getting tired after performing tasks that used to seem effortless. Many recently diagnosed with Parkinson's report that this is the effect they find most difficult to accept. Finding the time to rest is easier said than done, as is psychologically accepting the fact that you may need an afternoon nap. (See Month 8 for more information.)

Fatigue may be due to the physical stress of the disease, frustration with cognitive effects (having problems with concentration, having to think about tasks that used to be automatic, struggling to remember things), depression, or all of the above.

FREEZING

This means that all or part of your body is unable to move for a period of time—perhaps seconds, maybe several minutes. It seems to occur more frequently when walking through doorways or when turning around. (No one seems to know what it is about those particular movements that causes freezing.) These episodes can be very frightening as well as debilitating. About 30 percent of PD patients will experience freezing.[3]

Strategies for dealing with freezing

○ Visualize a line marking the door threshold and step over it. There are some walkers on the market now that can produce an infrared line that serves the same function.
○ March in place.
○ Count your steps.
○ Instruct your care partner and family members to give you a tap on the shoulder.
○ Some people with PD are now using service dogs to assist them with their daily activities. The dog can be taught to give you a nudge if it senses that you are "frozen."

HAND OR FOOT CRAMPS

Muscles that have been clenched for long periods of time tend to cramp. Many people with Parkinson's find that their toes or hands will curl up tightly. These cramps can be quite painful, and sometimes, if medication adjustments don't ease the problem, your physician may recommend physical therapy, massage therapy, or perhaps botox injections to temporarily relax the muscles.

LOSS OF HAND DEXTERITY

Separate from tremor, people with PD lose the ability to make many of the fine-motor movements that we unconsciously use all the time. Many newly diagnosed people report that this development was unexpected. Everyday tasks like buttoning a shirt or tying your shoes become difficult as Parkinson's disease progresses.

> I didn't realize that you lost dexterity, I thought you just shook. I was totally surprised by this. —MARY ANN, *diagnosed at 43*

Losing the ability to do tasks or enjoy hobbies that require fine, precise hand movements (tasks like surgery or assembly-line work; hobbies like woodworking, painting miniatures, bead-weaving) is also frustrating. If you are still working, it could mean the loss of your livelihood. But don't panic! In the workplace, accommodations can be made so you can do the same work with some assistance or you can be given a comparable task.

With hobbies, you may find that there are certain times of day that are better for doing the things that require controlled hand movements. You still have a window of opportunity to engage in your favorite hobbies but less time in which to do them.

LOSS OF FLUIDITY OF MOVEMENTS

Many Parkies have noted that one of their early symptoms was a loss of fluid or smooth movements. For example, raising an arm produced a ratcheting or cogwheeled, jerky effect. This symptom disappears with medication but unfortunately will come back to stay as the disease progresses.

It is possible to be slow and graceful, so if PD only affected the speed at which we do things, it wouldn't be so bad, but since we usually have rigidity as well, we become clumsy. Tools that were simple to use, such as salad tongs, can now become instruments of torture and humiliation if you are forced to use them when your medication is not working.

Tips for coping with loss of dexterity and/or fluidity

WE PARKIES are an adaptive, creative bunch. Here are just a few suggestions that you can use to maintain your independence in daily activities.

DRESSING

○ Whenever possible, wear shirts and pants that don't require any closures or fasteners: T-shirts or sweatshirts that can be slipped over your head, pants with elastic waistbands, pull-on skirts.

○ Choose shoes that slip on, have Velcro closures, or use curly shoestrings that don't need to be tied. (A list of some vendors of products like these is included in Resources.)

○ Use **assistive devices,** such as buttonhooks, zipper pulls, long-handled shoehorns, and the like. Occupational therapists have this type of information. Senior centers are another good source for obtaining product catalogs.

PERSONAL CARE

○ Use an electric toothbrush. Ask your dentist to recommend a brand. There are flossing devices on the market now that have long handles like a toothbrush; these make flossing back teeth much easier. If you get "dry mouth" from medications, proper brushing and flossing are especially important in order to avoid cavities. Regular dental visits are also important. If you think it's difficult to keep your mouth open to brush your teeth when your jaw is stiff, I can tell you from personal experience that holding your mouth open and your head still for a filling is much worse.

IN THE KITCHEN

○ Use utensils with ergonomic (designed for safety and ease of use) grips. Brands that are widely available in the housewares section of Target, Wal-Mart, hardware stores, and kitchen specialty shops include Oxo and Good Grips.

○ Rubber jar openers are useful, as are electric can openers.

○ Weighted silverware/flatware is easy to hold and provides better control for people who have tremors.

○ Special knives or cutting utensils, such as kitchen shears, are available and can make food preparation easier and safer.

○ Travel mugs with lids work well, even when you are not traveling. Do not fill mugs, glasses, or bowls more than half full, whenever possible. Ask for assistance if carrying plates and bowls, or accept help when it is offered.

○ Most wheeled walkers with seats have a tray attachment that assist you in moving heavy pots, pans, and so forth around the kitchen.

AROUND THE HOUSE

○ Use adapters for doorknobs, drawer pulls, lamp switches, and keys.

○ Check out the reaching devices that are available. They are much safer for you than standing on tiptoe or on a step stool to reach something.

ADMINISTRATIVE WORK

○ Use pens with thick rubber grips (these make the pen easier to hold). Consider getting a signature stamp for checks.

○ A handy hint for times when you need to fill in an address form: carry mailing labels with you. Many charities and businesses send them in the mail free-of-charge. This is a great use for them, and I know, in my case, they are much easier to read than my handwriting!

○ Get telephones and remote controls with large-button key pads. If you cannot find them, try to "test-drive" a product before you buy it. We recently bought a new cordless phone set, and I checked out the key pads on all models to assess how easy or difficult it was to press the keys and how likely I was to hit several keys at a time. I chose a model with a speakerphone feature in the handset as well as the base. This allows me to set the phone down and talk. Headsets can work well, too. These features keep my hands from cramping. It also means I don't try to use my shoulder to hold the phone against my ear.

○ Voice recognition software has come a long way, and though there is a bit of a learning curve, this type of product can be a godsend if you are having trouble typing. The translation mistakes it makes provide good entertainment, too.

MASKED FACE

It isn't physically painful as a rule (although clenched jaws are the exception), but loss of your facial expressions can affect your personal relationships, because people don't know how to "read" or interpret your expressions. Many people find that Sinemet helps to alleviate some masking, particularly in the first few years you take it.

STOOPED POSTURE

Rigid muscles in your neck and shoulders can pull your head down and your shoulders forward, giving you a stooped, humpback-like posture. To avoid this, get into a routine of stretching these areas daily.

LOSS OF BALANCE

Loss of balance is a common symptom of PD that can result in some nasty falls and can be made worse by certain medications. Here are some ways to avoid falling:

- ○ Slow down! I know that may seem silly since a hallmark of Parkinson's disease is slowed movements. However, knowing that I may have slow times during the day often makes me all the more likely to rush when I am "on." The times that I have fallen have been during those hurried moments.
- ○ Wear skid-resistant shoes or socks. "Hospital socks"—the fuzzy baby-blue things you get during a hospital a stay—are very handy. Slippers with nonskid treads are good for around the house.
- ○ Get up slowly. When you get out of bed, it's a good idea to sit up slowly, take a couple of seconds for your body to adjust, and then stand. If you go immediately from prone to standing too quickly, you may get dizzy or even faint.

"NO ONE TOLD ME IT COULD HURT!"

Muscle tension and rigidity hurt, especially when they have been going on for long periods of time. Shoulder pain is often an early sign of PD. It certainly was for me. Significant portions of the PD population (38 to 54 percent, depending on the study) feel pain that is related to their disease.[4] Forty percent of Parkinson's patients say that they have experienced numbness, tingling, and pain but when doctors investigate and find no so-called sensory deficits to back up a claim, they may discount the claim. Make sure that your physician is following the latest information on PD, which validates our reports of pain.

RESTRICTED BREATHING AND HYPERVENTILATION

I knew that muscle rigidity from PD could affect breathing, but until I began doing research for this book, I really had no idea how far-reaching the implications of that effect could be.

If your chest and diaphragm muscles are rigid, your lungs will not be able to take in as much air. Your breathing will be shallower and faster. If it becomes too rapid, it is called hyperventilation. Shallow breathing takes more energy, and you can become tired, which can lead to shortness of breath.

Some people with PD may develop a spinal deformity from prolonged muscle tension in the chest and diaphragm. (You may have seen some patients with advanced PD who have very stooped shoulders and appear to have a "hump.") If your spine becomes significantly affected, this may also reduce your breathing capacity. Dyskinesia, the involuntary movements that can result from long-term levodopa therapy, can also affect breathing.

Respiration is automatic, but proper breathing often requires conscious thought. Why is shallow breathing a big deal? Because if we do not take in enough oxygen, our brain and other organs do not get enough to function properly, which can result in confusion, memory problems, and anxiety. Waste products in the bloodstream will also not be flushed out completely. This can cause tingling in your hands and feet or around your mouth. It can cause blood vessels to contract, which could make your ears ring, and your vision to become blurred and make your hands and feet cold because the blood is not reaching them. Lastly, breathing affects the amount of energy our bodies use. Shallow breathing takes more energy, thereby burning more calories. But if we aren't getting enough oxygen, we may be too tired to eat. This can lead to a vicious cycle of fatigue, weight loss, depression, and anxiety.

SEXUAL DYSFUNCTION

Sex can be a taboo issue for many people, even if they don't have PD, and there has not been much research on how Parkinson's affects sex. What we do know is that men may experience erectile dysfunction, and women can have difficulty achieving orgasm. More information on sexual dysfunction and suggestions on coping can be found in Month 8.

SKIN PROBLEMS

You may feel like you are going through adolescence again—PD can make your skin very oily, especially on your face and scalp. The opposite problem—dry skin—can occur elsewhere on your body. Dandruff, eczema, and **seborrheic dermatitis** are common. Your doctor can prescribe skin care products that can control these conditions.

Do not use OTC cortisone creams, especially on your face, because long-term use can cause thinning of your skin.

Skin conditions can be an effect of PD, but they can also be signs that your autonomic nervous system (ANS) is not functioning properly. (The autonomic nervous system regulates all the unconscious but very necessary body functions, such as breathing, circulation, temperature control, and so on.) Problems with the ANS, combined with other symptoms, could indicate that you don't have idiopathic Parkinson's disease, and that you may have another form of parkinsonism. See page 38 in Day 3 for more information on other types of parkinsonism.

Both Parkinson's disease itself and some of the medications can cause excessive sweating. If at some point you find yourself covered with sweat when others in the room are comfortable, chances are that this is due to your PD.

PD can affect your body in many ways over the course of the illness. There are treatment methods for most of them, and remember, you won't experience each and every one.

IN A SENTENCE:

> As Parkinson's disease progresses, you may experience a variety of symptoms, including masking, cramping in your hands and feet, stooped posture, and shoulder and neck pain from muscle rigidity.

learning

Clognition— How Parkinson's Disease Can Affect You Mentally

IN DOING research for this book, I was surprised to find that some Finnish doctors whom I have never met could have me so well pegged. A study published in the 2001 *Proceedings of the National Academies of Science* begins, "For nearly a century, it has been suggested that Parkinson's disease could be associated with a specific personality type. The 'parkinsonian personality' has been described as compulsive, industrious, introverted, morally rigid, punctual, serious, stoic, and quiet."[5] Well, maybe not the "morally rigid" part, but the rest of the description fits me—and many other Parkies I know.

Obsessive-compulsive behavior

Many of us with PD have personalities that make us prone to addictions or **obsessive-compulsive behavior.** I have a history of eating disorders (anorexia and bulimia in high school and college). Those conditions have not been a problem in recent years, but I can still get very upset when I cannot control things. Of course, PD takes away my control over many aspects of my life now. Many of the other people with Parkinson's in my support group have experienced addiction to alcohol, drugs, gambling, sex, or shopping. Unfortunately, these traits can be made worse by dopamine agonists and Sinemet.[6] My husband can attest to my current addiction to radio contests and quizzes. This habit has been very lucrative—I've won concert tickets, DVDs, even a pair of video phones—but it is pretty pathetic that I have been known to arrange my day around my favorite radio stations' giveaways! Other Parkies have reported compulsions to paint, make jewelry, and chat online. Certainly, not all of these behaviors are harmful, but they do seem to support the claim that we tend to be compulsive.

Cognitive effects can cause identity crises

Most people—even many neurologists—think of Parkinson's as a purely physical disease, which we Parkies know is not the case. Researchers continue to discover cognitive effects associated with Parkinson's disease, such as memory problems, attention deficits (inability to focus on a task), and changes in executive function. "Executive function" refers to a person's "ability to anticipate, plan, initiate activities and inhibit [his/her] actions."[7] If you are like me and so many others with Parkinson's, you take your work very seriously. Feeling that you can't focus on your job or get things done in the timely, precise manner to which you are accustomed is not only frustrating; it can cause a crisis in confidence, a feeling that part of your identity is threatened.

These effects are very frustrating and disturbing, because they are so personal and they are invisible to others. When you experience tremors or are very stiff, other people are much more apt to understand that those symptoms are part of the disease. They are less likely to express empathy and support if you can't remember the reason you walked from one room to the next or can't concentrate on your work.

Worldwide Education and Awareness for Movement Disorders (WE MOVE) defines "cognition" as mental processes, including "perception, memory, awareness, reasoning, judgment, intellect, and imagination." Greg, a person with young-onset Parkinson's who was diagnosed at age forty-three, coined the term "clognition" to refer to the way that Parkinson's can affect our minds—the dense fog of depression, the clutter of obsessive or compulsive thoughts, and its veil of confusion. Scientists are just beginning to uncover the cognitive and mental impacts of physical symptoms that have been recognized for a long time.

Memory problems

PD affects our ability to remember things, but not in the same way as Alzheimer's disease. People with Parkinson's have trouble retrieving memories. When I think of literal examples of this in my own life, I see the large plastic storage box that is full of disparate papers, journals, and notes for this book. In a person with Alzheimer's disease, those memory files are actually missing.

Forgetfulness beyond that which is normally associated with age, impaired decision-making skills, and changes in our ability to process visual information are also part of the package of cognitive effects brought on by PD.

It is important to realize that a certain amount of forgetfulness comes with age, even if you don't have PD. That said, here are a few tips and tricks for dealing with memory issues:

○ "Use it or lose it." Keep your memory in shape by playing word games with your partner, kids, or grandchildren, doing crossword puzzles, or playing Trivial Pursuit with friends.

○ Mentally recite the ABCs backward or count backward from one hundred while brushing your teeth.

○ Make lists. When I get up each morning, one of the first things I do is make a list of things I need to do that day. I find that this early morning time is when I am best able to remember appointments or plans I've made. Just be sure to have a consistent place for keeping your list. Otherwise, you will discover, as I frequently do, that you have forgotten where you put it!

○ Assign words, mental images, or phrases to things that you need to remember. Examples are the common trick for remembering the musical notes on the lines of the treble clef ("Every Good Boy Does Fine"), or knowing which way to turn the wrench when changing a tire ("Right, tight. Left, loose.").

Confusion and mental fuzziness

In addition to forgetfulness, Parkinson's can also impair your decision-making skills and change your ability to process visual information. Parkinson's disease affects serotonin and norepinephrine levels as well as levels of dopamine. Serotonin is associated with alertness and consciousness. **Norepinephrine** (also known as **epinephrine, noradrenaline,** or **adrenaline,** just to add to your confusion) is involved in regulating mood. Thus, it should be no surprise that we can be cranky or overly emotional, confused, or forgetful.

Learn online

IF YOU want to learn more about the cognitive effects of PD, Carey Christensen, a forty-eight-year-old woman with Parkinson's, has a wonderful Web site called Clognition.org. It offers advice and information about PD's effects on cognition and features inspiring writing from many people with Parkinson's. Carey has made it her mission to educate physicians, care partners, and Parkies about the cognitive effects of the disease. She has also been a staunch advocate for more research and more support services for mental health issues associated with PD.

Braintalk (www.braintalk.org) also has an extensive list of online discussions on a very broad array of topics and problems, ranging from anger management to artistic expression to memory deficits. These discussions are a series of posted messages that are archived, so you can benefit from an experience that someone posted months ago, or you can search to find specific information.

Establish a baseline

One thing that you can do if you feel that the memory and cognitive problems you are experiencing are due to more than merely aging is to undergo a battery of tests to evaluate your cognitive functions. Your doctor may be willing to do these tests herself, or she may refer you to someone else. A variety of therapists are trained in this testing. For example, my testing was done by the speech therapist that my neurologist recommended. It is generally covered by insurance.

I actually thought the testing was fun. There were a variety of exercises, ranging from reciting lists of words or numbers, drawing pictures based on verbal and written instructions, to counting backward from one hundred by sevens. If at any time in the future, I am feeling worried or anxious that my cognitive abilities are really slipping, I can be retested and compare the results.

Dealing with anxiety

Anxiety is a common effect of PD. It is the general feeling that something bad could happen at any time, a "waiting for the other shoe to drop" sense of agitation or nervousness. Anxiety may cause us to overreact to normal everyday stressors, which can in turn make our PD symptoms worse. If our anxiety is not under control, then our bodies are in a constant state of trying to decide whether to fight or flee, leaving us vulnerable to colds and other illnesses on top of everything else.

There are a number of ways to deal with anxiety. They include guided imagery, relaxation techniques, meditation, counseling, and medication. Improper breathing techniques can produce anxiety, and conscious proper breathing can relieve it. Proper breathing is an integral part of several of these coping methods, especially relaxation techniques and meditation.

GUIDED IMAGERY

Guided imagery is based on the notion that seeing or thinking of particular scenes or objects can help you to relax or calm down and deal with anxiety-provoking incidents. For example, if you find yourself becoming anxious about going out in public because of your PD, you could practice visualizing a time before PD when you did a great job making a presentation or when you had a wonderful time dancing. Concentrate on remembering how good you felt at that time. Work on calling to mind the mental images and the feelings that you associate with them when you are feeling nervous about leaving the house.

There are many books, audiotapes, and videos available on guided imagery techniques. Many therapists also use the technique. You can check the Self-Help/Psychology section of your local bookstore or talk with a therapist about choosing the best images or situations to use for your own personalized guided imagery. You can record an audiotape or make a compact disc in which someone talks through the situation you should imagine or the images you should call to mind. Listen to this recording at bedtime or when you are feeling anxious. Pretty soon you will find that you can induce the calm, relaxed feeling without the recording.

RELAXATION TECHNIQUES

Relaxation techniques can involve music or audio instruction. For example, I have used a tape recording in which my therapist at the time instructed me to clench and then relax various parts of my body while soothing instrumental music played in the background. "Pull your toes up toward your body. Count to five. Then release. Experience the feeling of relaxation that has come into your toes." You move on up your body, keeping relaxed the areas you have already done. This is a good one to do at night when preparing for bed. Obviously, it is not one that you can do in a meeting or while driving to church. But it can be one effective "tool" in your "toolbox" of coping mechanisms.

MEDITATION

When many of us think of meditation, we picture someone sitting on a pillow, with their legs folded under them in some impossible position and chanting "Om." That is one way to meditate, and you can certainly go out and buy a *zafu* (one of the cushions you have probably seen people using when they meditate), but it is not the only way. You can meditate just as easily while sitting in a chair.

Meditation is sometimes defined as "clearing your mind" or "thinking about nothing." One of the goals of meditation is to get you to relax and stop focusing on the list of worries that is cluttering your mind. This is usually done by focusing your breathing, to the exclusion of everything else.

Many people meditate when they first wake up or right before bed. There are no magical times for meditation, and the primary space requirements are quiet and comfort. If you are like me and have a hard time doing nothing, meditation may be challenging for you, but I urge you to give it a try.

There are no "thought police" who will chastise you if you are unable to eliminate every single thought from your mind or if you cannot sit still for thirty minutes. I have found that when I make time to meditate, even if I am not doing it perfectly (i.e., sitting cross-legged and perfectly still on a *zafu* for an hour), I am calmer and more relaxed throughout the day.

Getting started can be difficult if you haven't attempted meditation before, but don't worry. There are plenty of ways to learn. If you would like to take a class or join a meditation group, contact your local community education programs, senior centers, retirement communities, alternative medicine centers, and the like.

Coping with the changes that PD brings to your mind and your body is definitely challenging, but the tools that I just mentioned can help you to get through tough spots. It is frustrating to feel that your identity, your purpose in life, is changing without your permission. But if you ignore the messages your body is sending, you are bringing on more stress, which exacerbates the situation. If you take time to relax and evaluate the situation, you may find a new purpose in life. And if you don't, being in a calmer mental state allows you to function more like your old self.

IN A SENTENCE:

> Forgetfulness, confusion, and mental fuzziness are some of the cognitive effects that may accompany your PD, but there are ways to deal with them.

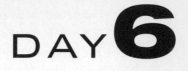

living

Depression and PD

AS YOU are coming to grips with your PD diagnosis, you may be feeling depressed. If so, you are not alone. Forty percent of people with Parkinson's get depressed at some point during their struggle with PD.[1]

Many of us were raised to associate depression or other mental health problems with character flaws or weakness. These attitudes can be difficult to overcome, particularly for men, who may think that therapy is okay for women but that males should be able to "pull themselves up by their own bootstraps."

Depression is an illness, not a sign of weakness

Doctors and other health-care providers now recognize that depression can be caused by physical changes in our individual body chemistries. Studies have shown that people who have experienced bouts of depression are more likely to later be diagnosed with depression. However, given the long latency period between when your dopamine-producing neurons begin to die and when PD is finally diagnosed, it could be that depression is an early symptom. Acccording to the National Institutes of Mental Health,

People with depression who have Parkinson's disease have a different symptom profile than those without Parkinson's. The Parkinson's profile includes higher rates of anxiety, sadness without guilt or self-blame, and lower suicide rates despite high rates of suicidal thoughts. Hormonal imbalances such as hypogonadism and hypothyroidism, which can cause depressive symptoms, need to be looked at carefully in these individuals. More research is needed to understand the relationship between Parkinson's disease and depression, dementia, anxiety disorders, and psychosis.[2]

I experienced my first bout of depression as a child and have had numerous encounters with it over the years, so now I can always tell when my brain chemistry has changed for the worse. The first time I sought treatment for depression was as a high school senior. I saw a psychologist who was very nice but unable to help me much, because I had decided that I would reveal my true feelings only if she asked exactly the right questions. She never did, and my depression went largely unchecked until I went through a treatment program for my eating disorders. It was there that a combination of talk therapy and antidepressant medication taught me that I didn't have to be miserable.

When I am depressed, I feel as if I am walking around with a wet wool blanket draped over me. I feel weighed down and trapped. All I want to do is eat, sleep, and cry. Things that I would normally enjoy are no fun. Since I am a very shy person anyway, others may not notice these changes. When I get "sick and tired of being sick and tired," I call a psychologist to make an appointment to talk, and I let her know which antidepressants have helped in the past. I have to work with a psychiatrist to get the right drug, which may take weeks, but now I know that I can be happy, even with Parkinson's, and I want to have that feeling back.

Depression is treatable

Depression is treatable for most people. You are not helping anyone by suffering in silence. In fact, by not seeking treatment for depression you can harm your relationship with family, friends, and coworkers. The stress of suffering from depression and anxiety can also make your PD symptoms worse. Having depression is nothing to be ashamed of. In fact, antidepressants are the first medications prescribed for many people when their Parkinson's disease is diagnosed.

It's normal but not inevitable to become depressed at the news that you are dealing with a chronic illness. Facing a progressive disease, having to retire or change jobs because of your illness, and moving because of your PD are just some of the very stressful experiences that you may experience in your journey with PD. It is normal to experience a sense of loss at such times, and grieving that loss is a very important part of healing.

If you aren't sure whether you are depressed, take a few minutes to review this list. If you are experiencing any of these symptoms, you may be depressed and would do well to consider seeing a therapist or counselor. It's also very common for care partners to experience bouts of depression. Caring for someone with PD presents many challenges, and all of these recommendations made for people with Parkinson's apply to care partners, too.

Symptoms of depression

- ○ Persistent sad, anxious, or "empty" mood
- ○ Feelings of hopelessness, pessimism
- ○ Feelings of guilt, worthlessness, helplessness
- ○ Loss of interest or pleasure in hobbies and activities that were once enjoyed, including sex
- ○ Decreased energy, fatigue, being "slowed down"
- ○ Difficulty concentrating, remembering, making decisions
- ○ Insomnia, early-morning awakening, or oversleeping
- ○ Appetite or weight loss, or overeating and weight gain
- ○ Thoughts of death or suicide; suicide attempts
- ○ Restlessness, irritability
- ○ Persistent physical symptoms that do not respond to treatment, such as headaches, digestive disorders, and chronic pain

If you've experienced five or more of these symptoms every day for at least two weeks and they interfere with routine daily activities such as work, self-care, and child care, or social life, seek an evaluation for depression.

Source: National Institutes of Mental Health.

Dealing with depression

Being depressed now does not mean that you are going to experience it for the rest of your life. Nor does it mean you'll always be on medication or have to endure years of weekly appointments at which you pour out your soul while lying on a couch as a bearded white male psychiatrist nods his head every so often. (That's a Woody Allen movie, not real life!)

Depression is not always treated with medication, but when it is, it's usually in combination with therapy. If you are prescribed medication, it's important to remember that antidepressants usually take weeks to become fully effective. Talking to someone, formally or informally, can help you get through that waiting period.

A few words of advice on confiding your feelings of depression: there is a long list of reasons why confiding solely to a family member or very close friend is not a good idea. It puts that person under a great deal of pressure to keep a secret. He may feel like he should "fix" the situation or that you expect him to do so. He will probably have a difficult time giving you objective feedback. Lastly, as someone close to you, he or she may also be experiencing feelings of depression around your PD. These are not meant as reasons to avoid discussing your feelings with friends and family. What I do mean, based on personal experience, is that having a "neutral observer's" point of view in addition to the views of your friends and family can be very beneficial for everyone.

Either in addition to medication or instead of it, your doctor may suggest you begin psychotherapy to address your depression. Psychotherapy means that you meet with a trained mental health professional, usually on a regular basis, to talk about your feelings. It does not have to go on for the rest of your life. Many people use weekly hourlong sessions for a few months and then go on an as-needed basis.

Your feelings of depression can be addressed in therapy in a number of ways, often using more than one of these therapeutic approaches.

For example, when a situation doesn't work out the way you would like, do you automatically assume that it is your fault, that you have done something wrong? Let's say you called a friend on Friday and left a message asking him to join you for dinner on Sunday. Now it's Monday morning and he still hasn't called. You have decided that he must be angry with you, and you spend the morning stewing about what you might have done. **Cognitive/**

behavior therapy would work with you to identify such patterns of thought and behavior and come up with other possibilities. Maybe your friend is out of town and hasn't even heard your message yet. Maybe his wife accidentally deleted the message as she was playing it back. Or maybe your friend was just really busy and forgot. Being aware of other realistic outcomes helps you to realize that you are not a bad person and that you do not control another person's feelings or actions.

Do you find that you feel anxious and stressed around your Aunt Mabel, which, in turn, makes your PD symptoms worse? The **interpersonal therapy** process would work with you to identify what it is about your relationship with your aunt that puts you in an anxious mood, with the theory that once you are aware of what it is about her that "pushes your buttons," you might be able to change the situation.

Speaking of Aunt Mabel, perhaps there was a specific event in your past that has haunted you over the years. Perhaps when you were six, you were having a tea party and broke several cups in her prized china tea service. She berated you for being clumsy and has called you "Clumsy Carol" ever since. **Psychodynamic therapy** would help you identify that incident from your past and try to help you deal with the shame and anxiety that you have about your PD tremors.

You do not necessarily have to see a psychiatrist or psychologist. Social workers and clergy members often receive counseling training as well. If you feel more comfortable talking to such a person, do so, but inquire first about any training they have had and any knowledge they have of PD issues. In addition, be aware that insurance is much more likely to pay for visits to a licensed counselor.

There's also group therapy, which is a structured support group. People with similar illnesses meet to discuss feelings and situations under the guidance of a facilitator. Members of the group give each other suggestions for coping, make observations about one another's behavior, and generally provide a forum where everyone can commiserate. Good support groups help their members acknowledge life's ups and downs and work through their feelings. This may happen in a "touchy-feely" sort of way, where group hugs are common, but such activities are not necessities for the success of the group.

If you don't know how to find a therapist or are concerned about how you will afford it, ask your doctor for a recommendation. You might also find it helpful to talk with your pastor/priest/rabbi/clergy member. If none of these options are useful to you, check your local phone listings for First Call for Help. This organization specializes in helping people to find community resources.

IN A SENTENCE:

> *Many people with Parkinson's experience depression—it's perfectly normal and very treatable.*

learning

Coming to Terms with Your Diagnosis

THE DAY you are diagnosed with Parkinson's disease will probably seem like the longest day of your life. From now on, coming to terms with your diagnosis will be an important factor in your mental health, which, in turn affects your disease. You will experience a number of emotions, ranging from anger and disbelief to worry and despair. You may feel a twinge of relief at finally having a diagnosis. You may feel alone in dealing with this news. I hope that this book will help you to avoid that feeling.

You are not alone

Being diagnosed with Parkinson's disease puts you in a group of more than one million Americans. This is not an elite club; it can affect anyone from any ethnic background, any social or economic stratum, either sex. Unfortunately, you do not get any door prizes for being chosen. I wish that I could provide you with a decoder ring to decipher the complex language of Parkinson's research documents, or a user's manual to tell you what to expect. You have already undergone the initiation rite by receiving your diagnosis. Your friends and family join an even larger club of people impacted by Parkinson's disease, because like any chronic disease or disability, it affects everyone, in ways we may not expect.

Whether your diagnosis with PD came like a sucker punch out of nowhere or as a long-awaited acknowledgment that there actually is something physically wrong with you and you are not merely "crazy," it is a stressful time.

The need to grieve

Sure, you may try to put on a brave face and say, "It could be worse." That is definitely true, and keeping a positive attitude is critical as part of a plan to minimize the progression of your disease. But even the most optimistic person will have moments when she needs to grieve for everything that Parkinson's disease will take away from her.

I have heard therapists talk about the need to grieve over the losses that PD has caused or will cause in your life, just as you would grieve over the loss of a loved one. Indeed, we are all dealing with the "death" of hopes, dreams, and plans. New hopes, dreams, and plans can take their place, but only after we have made peace with what we have lost.

Care partners and family members experience grief, too

All of this holds true for care partners and family members, too—not just the person with PD. In fact, care partners experience a greater amount of guilt, because they find themselves being angry with their partner for ruining their plans for the future, taking up their free time, receiving all the attention, and so on.

In her 1969 pioneering book, *Death & Dying*, psychiatrist Elizabeth Kübler-Ross theorized that grief comes in five stages: denial; anger/resentment; bargaining; depression; and acceptance. With all due respect to Dr. Kübler-Ross's work, I think that the emotions identified are definitely involved, but use of the term "stages" implies a linear progression—that you start at one end and work your way through to the other. In my experience, grief is more like a maze. You think you've found your way to the point where you have made it through to the doorway of acceptance. Then you make a wrong turn and suddenly you are back at the beginning, lost in denial. So I am going to address these emotions as rooms in what I call "the grieving maze."

THE DENIAL ROOM

I think that it's safe to say that virtually everyone, upon hearing the words "I think you have Parkinson's disease," does the emotional equivalent of rushing into this room and slamming the door. We need a warm, dark cocoon in which we can escape and calm ourselves. We may chant a mantra like "This isn't happening. This cannot be happening." In the denial room, we cut ourselves off from anything that we don't want to hear. I suppose in that sense, this could also be called the "control room," since it is where we try to exert control over what we feel and do not feel.

Denial is normal and healthy—to a point. Some people dwell in the denial room for a long time. Even when you do venture out into the other parts of the maze, a new symptom or situation may put you right back there. For instance, I was in denial for years about how my disease was affecting my ability to do my job. My body proceeded to make it very obvious, to the point that I could no longer ignore it. It took a trip to the emergency room because of chest pains to get the point across that I was indeed under too much stress.

THE ANGRY ROOM

Obviously, it is normal to be angry when you receive a diagnosis of PD. The important thing is to experience that anger and get past it. In my opinion, if we surrender to anger and allow it to affect everything we do, then the disease wins. And I don't think any of us want that.

For this emotion, it may be helpful to have a real physical space and time when you allow yourself to express your anger. Maybe it is a spare bedroom or office where you can scream, punch pillows, throw things; maybe it is a secluded area outdoors where you can throw rocks into a pond or stamp your feet. It may be in your car during a daily commute. (I have found screaming at the top of my lungs while driving to be very therapeutic, although it probably looks rather silly to anyone passing by.) Do whatever it takes to help you feel better. Just be careful not to hurt yourself or anyone else!

THE BARGAINING ROOM

This is where deals are made—often with God or a higher power, but also with a care partner, family member, even yourself. You may be thinking "God, if you would make it so that I don't have Parkinson's disease, I promise that I will. . . ." That blank may be "stop drinking," "start exercising," "spend more time with my family," "attend church every Sunday"—whatever offer you think would make God happiest. You may even make good on some of your promises, but I believe that most people move on from this room pretty quickly when they realize their prayers have not been answered.

THE DEPRESSION ROOM

When being angry or proposing deals does not work, it is very easy and normal to get depressed. This depression can be what is called "exogenous depression," meaning that it is a response to a situation rather than a chemical imbalance. Or the ineffectiveness of your anger and bargaining may amplify existing depression.

To me, this room feels like it is full of tar or quicksand. Everything feels very heavy, and making any movement toward the door takes a great deal of effort and commitment. This is another room in which it is easy to spend a great deal of time. If you do not have a history of clinical depression, you might spend only a few days or weeks here. If you have been depressed before, it could be a matter of months. You are apt to spend less time being depressed if you seek help in dealing with your situation.

THE ACCEPTANCE ROOM

Getting to this place, even if you don't stay there forever, will give your emotional and physical being the chance to restore itself. This is important, because dealing with the other emotions is very draining and stressful, which, in turn, exacerbates the symptoms of PD. Acceptance does not mean surrendering yourself to the disease. It means that you are being honest with yourself, being realistic about what you can and cannot do. I believe that acceptance means learning to take care of myself first so that I have the energy and the will to help others. Selfishness and self-preservation are not the same thing.

Going in circles

I have experienced at least those five emotions many times since I was diagnosed in 1998, although by the time I actually got a diagnosis, I think I was past denying that I had PD. Now I struggle with denying that I need to slow down, to ask for help. The following quote by Leo C. Rosten has been a guiding force in my life since I discovered it while doing research for a political psychology class:

> I think the purpose of life is to be useful, to be responsible, to be honorable, to be compassionate. It is, after all, to matter: to count, to stand for something, to have made some difference that you lived at all. —LEO C. ROSTEN, as quoted in *Living, Loving & Learning*. Leo F. Buscaglia, PhD. New York: Fawcett Columbine, 1982, 37.

I used to think that this meant getting through life by being a leader, blazing a clear trail for others to follow. Now I am beginning to realize that there are many ways that one can be a leader, and that in each room of the grieving maze and in each trip through it, I interact with people. I can make much more of a difference and be more useful if the path left by my life looks like a Spirograph design.

Other common emotions

The above five emotions are not the only ones you are likely to encounter during your grieving process. Here are a few others you may recognize:

Panic. This is that "Oh my gosh, I don't know how I'm going to cope" stage, where you think about all the things you still want to do with your life and wonder if you're going to have time to do them.

Guilt. You may start thinking things like "What have I done to my family?" and "If only I hadn't [done _____]." Guilt is anger turned inward, and we use that anger to try to beat ourselves into submission or as punishment for real or imagined transgressions.

Hostility. You may find yourself feeling anger and resentment toward people around you who are healthy.

Paralysis. Sometimes people become emotionally paralyzed, unable to resume activities because of their mental state.

Faith or hope. To me, an act of faith is when a person gets out of bed in the morning and puts down her feet, trusting that the floor will be there even if she cannot see it. There are different belief systems about who is responsible for the floor being there, but the action is the same.

I think that hope is more timid; a hopeful person may only extend one foot off the bed to probe the darkness. Yet that willingness to take that risk is what keeps us alive.

If you have neither faith nor hope, you surrender your identity to the disease. Although it may sound trite right now, your life will go on, and you can still have a lot of love and joy in your life.

Numerous self-help books are available to help you and your family deal with the losses and changes that PD will bring to your life. One that I have found beneficial is *Awakening from Grief* by John E. Welshons.

Hope is the adrenaline of the soul. —AMY TAN, *The Opposite of Fate: A Book of Musings*

Advice from others dealing with PD

Parkies and care partners had a variety of responses to my survey question about the best advice for the newly diagnosed, but there were some common themes, which I have incorporated into a mnemonic to make it easier to remember. It is the IDEAL way to cope with your first year of PD: individuality, drugs, exercise, attitude, and learning.

Individuality. Keep in mind that Parkinson's disease affects everyone differently within a range of symptoms. Focus on the positive aspects of this. You will not develop every symptom, and the rate of progression will be unique to you. If you see another person with PD who is in rough shape, do not assume that this will happen to you.

Drugs. Medications will be an important component of your treatment program as your disease progresses. This decision is one that you and your doctor should make together.

Exercise. Almost everyone stressed the importance of getting into a regular exercise routine. Many people said they wished they had realized the long-term impact that exercise can have on your prognosis and the progress of the disease.

Attitude. Your approach to life is critical. My friend Jack, who was diagnosed at age fifty, said these words of wisdom came "from my therapist, when I asked for advice on dealing with chronic illness: 'Make a place for it in your life. Then keep it in its place.' For me that meant to do what I needed to do regarding medications, sleep, exercise, etc., but then live my life as fully as possible. To not become the disease."

Learning. Learn everything you can about Parkinson's disease.

IN A SENTENCE:

> *Coming to terms with your disease involves many emotions, and you will most likely experience them more than once during your journey with PD.*

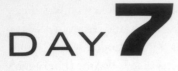

DAY 7

living

Telling Your Friends and Family

I KNOW that in the beginning you are still coming to terms with your own feelings about the overwhelming news that you have just received. Having to deal with it alone, combined with the stress of trying to cover up any visible symptoms, may only make things worse.

Telling loved ones is never easy

Telling loved ones that you have a chronic illness is never easy. However, it is very likely that close friends and family members have already noticed that something is going on. Many people report that when they finally mustered the courage to tell a family member or friend that they have Parkinson's disease, the person responded with a certain degree of relief, because PD isn't a terminal illness. Pam, who was diagnosed more than eight years ago, at the age of thirty-eight, recommends that you "don't try to hide it—let your friends and relatives know that you have PD. It's natural to want to hide it or to be in denial—especially if you're a person with young-onset PD. But hiding it adds to the stress."

Whenever possible, tell people individually or in very small groups. Doing so shows the people involved that you care about them and will allow you to get personal support.

Deciding when to tell people is entirely up to you, and much of it depends on the severity of your symptoms, the amount of contact you have with the person in question, and whether she knows you have been experiencing health problems. One thing you might want to think about is how you would feel in her position. Would you prefer to hear the news from her directly? Or would it be easier if someone else told you? (I think that most of us would choose to hear the news from a friend rather than through the grapevine.)

Timing is important

Try to choose a time when everyone involved will be available to really talk about the situation and comfort one another, ask and answer questions, and deal with the grief that your disclosure will bring. As tempting as it may be to wait until the good-byes at the airport after a holiday visit to say, "Oh, by the way, I just found out I have Parkinson's disease. Gotta go," doing so will not make the situation easier.

You set the tone

People will generally take their cues about how to react and how to treat you in the future from your attitude when you break the news. If they sense that you are ashamed of having PD or are embarrassed about it, they will be much less likely to inquire about your condition as it progresses. They may exclude you from activities—not necessarily because they don't want you there but because they think that even asking you will put you in an awkward position. For those of you who have participated in any Twelve-Step programs (Alcoholics Anonymous, Alanon, etc.), this situation is like "the elephant in the living room" that no one wants to approach.

Help is on the way

Prepare yourself for offers of help. Loved ones feel powerless when someone they are close to gets sick or hurt. Finding a way to let your friends and family help you is a way to show that you value their love and support. That help may come in the form of sending you every news story in the local paper that mentions PD or pointing out every ad for a "miracle cure" from supermarket tabloids. If that sort of thing drives you crazy, you have a couple of options: tell Aunt Mary, or your nephew George, or Elsie from your church group that you appreciate their information but you are already under a doctor's care, thanks anyway. Or you can take their information with a smile and recycle it as soon as they are out of sight. The most honest response, and thus usually the most difficult, is to say, "You know, what I really need from you is . . ." and actually tell them how they could be most supportive. That may be a hug, a shoulder to cry on, or a conversation about something other than PD.

Holly, a care partner whose husband was diagnosed at age forty-six, expressed regret that she and her husband had followed the doctor's advice, because she realized that by doing so they had unintentionally taken away their loved ones' opportunities to feel that they were being helpful and showing their love.

> Our diagnosing MD told us to "live our lives" as though we
> had not received the diagnosis and to discourage others
> from sending us every new treatment they heard of, etc.
> We followed his advice, and I feel this was very hard on
> family and friends. Information was a way . . . the only way
> they had to help and show they cared. This way of "pre-
> tending" didn't help anyone, as far as I can tell, and to this
> day, friends and family are confused as to how much they
> can say or ask us.

You do not have to go into this situation unprepared. I hope that in this section of the book, you will find encouragement and strength to decide which methods may work best for telling your loved ones about your PD. Acknowledge that your life has changed.

Parkinson's disease will affect how fast and how easily you can do the things you have always done. It is not helpful to pretend that you haven't changed, as Mary, who was diagnosed at fifty-three, discovered when dealing with her family.

> I tried so hard to ignore the whole thing that I painted
> myself into a corner and had to announce that I was not
> as I used to be and I couldn't do things. People are so care-
> ful about pretending you are "normal," and as I find more
> things that I can't do, it gets harder to work into the
> conversation.

A person newly diagnosed with PD must decide which and how many
people he or she is going to tell.

> In my case, I immediately told my inner circle of friends
> whom I knew would support me. I also took a risk and told
> my immediate supervisor (the principal) at school. I always
> felt that if I had no control over this disease, I could at least
> control the dispensing of the news. After a year, I told
> everyone else whom I felt was significant in my life and
> whom I didn't want to find out any other way. Entering the
> third year, I basically put it out there for anyone in my
> world. I wanted them to know why I walked the way I did,
> etc. There are still a lot of people who are marginally "in
> my world" and I don't care if they know or not. —MATT,
> *diagnosed at 49*

Be prepared

For many of the people you tell, you will be the first person they know
who is dealing with early stages of the disease, and they are likely to have
many questions. By having some printed information or resources available to offer them, you can educate them about the disease. Don't make
them accept it, but do offer it. Perhaps you can read it together and discuss it.

Your doctor's office may have pamphlets or brochures about PD. All of
the national Parkinson's organizations have a variety of informational materials that are available free of charge. You will find contact information for
those groups in the Resources section.

Put it in writing

Sometimes it's preferable or necessary to tell someone in writing—for example, if you are going to attend a wedding where you will be seeing many relatives whom you haven't seen in years. If you have obvious symptoms, such as a tremor, you might decide to write a short note to those whom you want to hear the news from you. Something like:

> Dear Aunt Mary,
>
> I am looking forward to seeing you at Cousin Mike's upcoming wedding. It will be an exciting occasion. I wanted to let you know that my life has changed a lot since the last time I saw you.
>
> I have been diagnosed with Parkinson's disease, a progressive neurological disease that can affect my body in many ways. When you see me, you may notice that [give an example: I have a tremor in my left hand; I drag my right foot when I walk; my voice is much softer than it used to be]. It is important to me to be the one to tell you this— not because I want your sympathy or to cause you to worry. On the contrary, I want to let you know that this is not fatal or contagious, and that I am being treated to minimize my symptoms.
>
> Let's keep this wedding a day to celebrate Cousin Mike's marriage to Jennifer, not a pity party for me. If you have any questions about Parkinson's disease or how I am doing, please feel free to ask me.
>
> See you soon!
>
> Love,
>
> Matthew

Telling casual acquaintances and neighbors

You have much more leeway when deciding whether to tell the person next door or someone you see occasionally at church. You have much more control over the timing and the manner in which you break the news, so don't force yourself to tell everyone at once. In some ways, it is much easier to tell people who are not related to you. If it doesn't go well, you can avoid them.

Why tell nonfamily members?

Maybe this is just "Minnesota nice," but here we make sure our next-door neighbors have a key to our house, in case of emergencies. When I had my "wake-up call" with the chest pains, I called 911 and my neighbor was able to lock up my house while I rode in the ambulance. I was mortified that I had to call her, but it gave me one less thing to worry about. Neighbors in particular can be very helpful if you find yourself in need of assistance.

With more than one million people with Parkinson's disease in this country, you don't have to go very far before you meet someone who knows someone with PD. You would be surprised how common it is to hear, "Yeah, my great-uncle had that" or "My minister has PD." Being open about your disease can actually put you in touch with support and resources that you otherwise would not have.

Dealing with rejection

If denial of the problem is the response that you get from some of those you tell, try to remember that their reaction is likely their way of handling the pain they feel when watching someone they love experience a disease. For many of our friends and loved ones, it is just too difficult to bring up the subject of PD. Some may go so far as to avoid contact with you because of the discomfort they experience. This is very sad, but as with so many things in life, we can't control the behavior of others.

A member of my support group tells a heartbreaking story about his grandchildren refusing to hold his hand because of his severe tremors. Unfortunately, this sort of rejection can occur. As we educate others about Parkinson's disease, hopefully such behavior will disappear. In the meantime, it can make coping very difficult.

If people you love are in denial about your disease, I would suggest not pushing them. Encourage them to attend support group meetings or come along to doctor appointments, and offer to answer any questions that they may have.

The question we all dread: "How ARE you?"

I am convinced that this single question is the primary reason that we dread telling others about our illness. It can be such a loaded question, and we can be so paranoid. I know that on "bad" days, when I am depressed or crabby or my meds aren't working, this simple inquiry can set off a cascade of self-criticism and self-pity. I find myself thinking, "Gee, do I look that bad? Does he really want to know how I'm doing? Will she ever ask me again if I give an honest response?" The flip side of that paranoia can be, "I know that she/he is thinking, 'He isn't shaking. I'll bet he doesn't have Parkinson's at all. Maybe he is just trying to get attention.'"

I will not pretend to have a universal solution to dealing with this question. All I can say is that I try to give people the benefit of the doubt and assume that they are genuinely concerned about my well-being and that they understand that I am not my disease. If they wanted to know how well I am coping with my disease, they would have asked that. By responding about how I am, I can reinforce for all of us that my life is not "all Parkinson's, all the time."

If you find yourself getting annoyed with family members or friends who seem to be always asking about your PD, take a moment to think about how you respond to their inquiries. I know that in some of my own interactions, I have been part of the problem because I've assumed someone was asking about my PD and I responded to that. I am getting better at telling someone how Jackie is doing. Then if they ask, "No, really, how are you?" I can respond, "Oh, do you mean how is my PD?" and take it from there.

IN A SENTENCE:

> *These tips and anecdotes can be helpful as you consider when and how to tell your family and friends about your Parkinson's disease diagnosis.*

learning

Drug Therapy for Depression and Anxiety

IF YOUR doctor does recommend antidepressants to help you deal with the anxiety or depression that may accompany your PD, especially in this early period while you are coming to terms with your diagnosis, there are some things that you should know. Any time there are any changes in your brain chemistry, you are apt to experience some unexpected repercussions, because there is still so much that medical science does not know about the brain.

Here is a list of some of the drugs most commonly prescribed for anxiety and depression in people with PD. Please be aware that your doctor may choose a medication that is not listed here if she feels it is better suited to your situation.

Some Common Medications for Depression and Anxiety*

Drug/ Brand Name	Type of Medication	Symptoms Treated	Side Effects
Buproprion (Wellbutrin®)	Antidepressant	Depression, withdrawal symptoms of smoking	Changes in weight or appetite, decreased sex drive, diarrhea, difficulty achieving orgasm, dizziness, dry mouth, frequent urination, flulike symptoms (muscle aches, discomfort, fatigue), headache, impotence, insomnia, nausea, nervousness, ringing in the ears, skin rash, sweating, tremor
Alprazolam (Xanax®)	Benzodiazepine	Anxiety, panic attacks	Behavior changes, clumsiness, decreased sex drive, depression, difficulty urinating, dizziness, drowsiness, dry mouth, GI problems (constipation, diarrhea, nausea, vomiting), headache, vivid dreams. Can by physically and psychologically addicting.
Buspirone (Buspar®)**	Anti-anxiety	Anxiety	Drowsiness, dry mouth, nightmares or vivid dreams
Citalopram (Celexa®)**	Selective serotonin reuptake inhibitor (SSRI)	Depression	Changes in weight or appetite, decreased sex drive, diarrhea, difficulty achieving orgasm, dizziness, dry mouth, headache, impotence, insomnia, nausea, nervousness, tremor
Diazepam (Valium®)	Benzodiazepine	Anxiety, muscle spasms	Behavior changes, clumsiness, decreased sex drive, depression, difficulty urinating, dizziness, drowsiness, dry mouth, GI problems (constipation, diarrhea, nausea, vomiting), headache, vivid dreams. Can by physically and psychologically addicting.

Drug/ Brand Name	Type of Medication	Symptoms Treated	Side Effects
Escitalopram (Lexapro®)**	SSRI	Depression, anxiety	Changes in weight or appetite, decreased sex drive, diarrhea, difficulty achieving orgasm, dizziness, dry mouth, headache, impotence, insomnia, nausea, nervousness, tremor
Fluoxetine (Prozac®)**	SSRI	Depression, obsessive-compulsive disorder (OCD), panic attacks, premenstrual syndrome	Changes in weight or appetite, decreased sex drive, diarrhea, difficulty achieving orgasm, difficulty concentrating, dizziness, dry mouth, excessive sweating, headache, impotence, insomnia, nausea, nervousness, tremor, weakness
Fluvoxamine (Luvox®)**	SSRI	Obsessive-compulsive disorders (OCD)	Changes in weight or appetite, decreased sex drive, diarrhea, difficulty achieving orgasm, dizziness, dry mouth, headache, impotence, insomnia, nausea, nervousness, tremor
Lorazepam (Ativan®)	Benzodiazepine	Anxiety	Behavior changes, clumsiness, decreased sex drive, depression, difficulty urinating, dizziness, drowsiness, dry mouth, GI problems (constipation, diarrhea, nausea, vomiting), headache, vivid dreams. Can by physically and psychologically addicting.
Mirtazapine (Remeron®)	Antidepressant	Depression	Constipation, dizziness, drowsiness, dry mouth, increased appetite/weight, nausea, tremor
Paroxetine (Paxil®)**	SSRI	Depression, anxiety, obsessive-compulsive disorder (OCD), panic attacks, posttraumatic stress disorder (PSTD), premenstrual syndrome, social anxiety	Changes in weight or appetite, decreased sex drive, diarrhea, difficulty achieving orgasm, dizziness, dry mouth, headache, impotence, insomnia, nausea, nervousness, tremor

Drug/ Brand Name	Type of Medication	Symptoms Treated	Side Effects
Sertaline (Zoloft®)**	SSRI	Depression, anxiety, obsessive-compulsive disorder (OCD), panic attacks, post-traumatic stress disorder (PSTD), premenstrual syndrome, social anxiety	Changes in weight or appetite, decreased sex drive, diarrhea, difficulty achieving orgasm, dizziness, dry mouth, headache, impotence, insomnia, nausea, nervousness, tremor
Venlafaxine (Effexor®)	Antidepressant	Depression, anxiety, social anxiety	Abnormal dreams, anxiety, dizziness or drowsiness, GI effects (nausea, vomiting, abdominal pain, weight loss), increased blood cholesterol, insomnia, sexual effects (decreased sex drive, impotence, abnormal ejaculation, difficulty achieving orgasm), sweating, yawning

* This list was derived from responses to my survey, conversations with other people with Parkinson's and care partners, and conversations and written materials from my neurologist and psychiatrist. It is not intended to reflect the pharmaceutical universe of options for treating depression and anxiety.

** If you are on Selegiline or rasagiline with these medications, be sure to thoroughly discuss the dosage and timing of all medications. Severe reactions are possible with these combinations of drugs.

Side effects of antidepressant medications

Antidepressants can offer considerable relief from feelings of anxiety, apathy, and feeling overwhelmed. However, there may be side effects associated with that relief.

Some common side effects associated with antidepressants include nausea, vomiting, loss of appetite, headache, insomnia, dizziness, dry mouth, sexual dysfunction, and weight gain. All antidepressants warn about the risks of drinking alcohol while you are on the medication. Excessive drinking can cause seizures.

It's worth noting that all antidepressants are required to be labeled with the following warning, which was decreed after evidence emerged that many antidepressants were linked to increased suicidal tendencies in children and teens taking the medications.

> While you are taking _____, you may need to be monitored for worsening symptoms of depression and/or suicidal thoughts especially at the start of therapy or when doses are changed. Your doctor may want you to monitor for the following symptoms: anxiety, panic attacks, difficulty sleeping, irritability, hostility, impulsivity, severe restlessness, and mania (mental and/or physical hyperactivity). These symptoms may be associated with development of worsening symptoms of depression and/or suicidal thoughts or actions. Contact your health-care provider if you develop any new or worsening mental health symptoms during treatment with _____. Do not stop taking _____ without first talking to your health-care provider.

Everyone has his or her own body chemistry that reacts differently to medication. You may experience some of these effects or none at all. You may experience an effect not listed. This is why it is important to pay close attention to your body when you begin a new medication. It is helpful to keep a diary of your medication intake anyway, since your doctor will most likely ask you at each visit how things are going.

IN A SENTENCE:

> *Depression is associated with Parkinson's disease, although it's unclear if it is generally a symptom or the result of the condition.*

FIRST-WEEK MILESTONE

I know that this first week has been a tough one, but you have learned a lot that will help you to deal with your personal journey with Parkinson's disease.

○ YOU HAVE LEARNED THAT THERE ARE FOUR PRIMARY SYMPTOMS OF PD BUT THAT NOT EVERYONE HAS ALL FOUR OR TO THE SAME DEGREE.

○ YOU KNOW THAT WHEN YOU AND YOUR DOCTOR DECIDE THAT YOU NEED THEM, THERE ARE MANY MEDICATIONS THAT CAN TREAT YOUR SYMPTOMS.

○ YOU HAVE INFORMATION ABOUT DEALING WITH DEPRESSION, WHICH YOU MAY EXPERIENCE AS A COMMON PART OF THE DISEASE.

○ YOU REALIZE THAT THE CAUSE OF PD IS NOT KNOWN, AND THAT NO CONSCIOUS ACT ON YOUR PART HAS CAUSED THE DISEASE.

Complementary Therapies

THERE ARE many complementary therapies—treatments that are given in addition to, not in place of, drug therapy—for PD. What follows is not an exhaustive list. I am including only the ones that are widely available at this time and for which there is substantial published, peer-reviewed evidence that the therapy might be helpful. I have specifically not included therapies that advocate discontinuation of levodopa therapy. Surgery and stem cell therapy are addressed separately. For all of the therapies mentioned in this section, you should at least let your health-care provider know that you intend to pursue them. When taking any vitamins, minerals, or herbal substances, check with a pharmacist who is well versed in those products, not just in pharmaceuticals.

> I would have liked to have had access to doctors and therapies that were more natural and holistic. The mainstream docs discouraged our seeking them out, but when we found the right MD, my husband's symptoms improved and he didn't experience the reactions of on/off or cognition/alertness difficulties so often reported.
> —HOLLY, *a care partner whose husband was diagnosed at 48*

Acupuncture

For more than 3,000 years, this ancient Chinese practice has been used to treat a wide array of physical and mental ailments. Very fine needles (a bit thicker than a human hair) are inserted into some of the 365 points on your body that correlate to specific organs or areas. The insertion points are located on a vast network of energy channels or meridians. These meridians are part of the system that distributes **chi** (pronounced "chee"), the Chinese word for "energy," throughout your body. **Acupuncture** and other Eastern medical traditions are based on the belief that when chi is blocked or impeded somewhere within the body, the blockage will manifest itself as an illness or health condition. Acupuncture uses needles to open the meridians and allow energy to flow freely. Medical experts who practice Western medicine—that is, the kind that strives to prove the cause of an illness or condition using scientific methods, risk assessments, and mathematical models—remain baffled about how acupuncture works. However, a literature review on the peer-reviewed medical Web site Medscape reported that a panel convened by NIH has concluded that there is scientific evidence that acupuncture can treat nausea and vomiting effectively. The American Academy of Medical Acupuncture has found that acupuncture can be helpful in treating pain, muscle spasms, **parasthesias** (tingling sensations), "frozen shoulder," and anxiety, among other health conditions.[1] While PD is not mentioned specifically, all of these problems can occur as part of the Parkinson's experience. I have received acupuncture from several different providers in Chicago, Seattle, and Minneapolis and found it to be helpful for muscle stiffness.

Some Western physicians have received acupuncture training in additional to their medical training, as have numerous chiropractors. People who study acupuncture without prior medical training must complete hundreds of hours of training and have proof of this (a diploma or certificate from a reputable institution) and a license. The National Certification Commission for Acupuncture and Oriental Medicine (www.nccaom.org) can provide a listing of licensed acupuncturists if your doctor cannot recommend one.

Traditional Chinese medicine

Acupuncture may be used in conjunction with traditional Chinese medicine (TCM). TCM uses herbs and other natural substances to produce remedies.

The key principle in traditional Chinese medicine is that both wellness and illness result from an imbalance of yin and yang. Yin refers to the feminine aspect of life: nourishing, lower, cool, deficient, inside, receptive, protective, soft, yielding. Yang is the male counterpoint: hard, dominant, energetic, upper, hot, excessive, outside, creative. The movement between these opposite forces, chi, is considered to be the essential element in the healing system of TCM.[2]

If you want to try TCM remedies and are currently taking conventional prescription drugs, you will need to involve your health-care provider and pharmacist. Also, be certain that the TCM practitioner understands that you are taking prescription medications. Ask about known or possible interactions. Unfortunately, there has not been much research about interactions between pharmaceuticals and herbal remedies. Herbs and vitamin/mineral substances are not subject to regulation by the Food and Drug Administration (FDA), so quality control and uniformity of dosages could be a problem.

Massage

Some people think that getting a massage means getting a backrub. Or they may be under the impression that the word is merely a euphemism for an illicit sex act. Licensed massage therapists do refer to their vocation as "bodywork," but they do not mean this in a sexual context.

A good massage will leave you very relaxed. You may also be drowsy. Massage has been shown to relieve muscle rigidity associated with PD. It may also help to reduce other symptoms by helping your body deal with stress. Massage therapy improves blood circulation and encourages your muscles and organs to release toxins that have built up in your body. Drinking plenty of water for the rest of the day after you have had a massage will flush those impurities from your system.

There are several types of massage, and licensed practitioners are required to undergo considerable training and pass an exam. Therapists who have achieved this status will list the initials LMT after their name. This stands for "licensed massage therapist." Some states do not require licenses. In that case, look for an individual who is a certified massage therapist (CMT), meaning that he or she has completed a training program at a massage school.

TYPES OF MASSAGE

Shiatsu means "finger pressure" in Japanese. A seven-year-old boy started the practice in 1912 in Japan. He applied finger pressure to certain areas of his mother's body to help alleviate the pain caused by her arthritis.[3] A shiatsu practitioner uses her hands to apply pressure to certain areas on your body. These areas correlate to the same meridians, or "energy channels," used in acupuncture. It is usually done fully clothed, and you will lie on a cot or massage table.

Watsu is a recently created combination of water exercise and shiatsu. As in shiatsu, a therapist will work on pressure points on your body. She will also guide your limbs through gentle stretches. This is done in a warm-water pool rather than on a massage table. Because it does involve massage, it is covered by most insurance companies.

Swedish massage is a "collection of techniques designed primarily to relax muscles by applying pressure to them against deeper muscles and bones, and rubbing in the same direction as the flow of blood returning to the heart."[4] Practitioners claim that Swedish massage stimulates your skin and the circulation of blood throughout your body as it relaxes your muscles and rids them of lactic acid. (Lactic acid is a waste product that builds up in muscles when they are strained.)

Typically, you remove all of your clothing except your underwear for this type of massage. (Some massage therapists provide hospital-style gowns for clients to wear.) Your body will be covered by a blanket or sheet so you are not exposed and to keep you warm. The massage therapist will fold back the sheet from the body part he is working on (i.e., your leg, arm, or back) and use a lotion or an oil to prevent friction when rubbing your skin. Sometimes the oil or lotion will have a scent (not that many of us with PD would notice this), so if you are sensitive or allergic to any fragrance products, let the therapist know before he begins the massage.

Deep-tissue massage is often used to loosen up the rigid muscles that we Parkies tend to have. It involves deeper, stronger pressure than other types of massage and muscles may be rubbed "against the grain." As is the case with Swedish massage, you will remove your clothes. Lotions or oils are used to lubricate your skin. This technique may result in some muscle soreness after the massage. Ice packs (or unopened bags of frozen vegetables) and OTC pain relievers can help with that.

I am a big fan of deep-tissue massage and have seen several massage therapists over the years, even before being diagnosed with PD. I have found that deep-tissue massage works well to reduce the "knots" of muscle that form in my neck and shoulders when I am under a lot of stress. Some insurance plans will cover deep-tissue massage therapy, so be sure to check with yours before you make an appointment. They may require a referral from your doctor.

Tai chi

Tai chi ("TIE chee") is an ancient Chinese combination of self-defense and exercise. It involves the use of gentle physical movement with mental imagery and breathing. The names for the motions are taken from nature, such as "wave hands like clouds."

Tai chi's influence on balance seems to greatly reduce our risk of falling. Researchers at Emory University in Atlanta, Georgia noted a 40 percent reduction in falls among elderly patients who practiced tai chi. Having better balance can be a big confidence booster!

Tai chi is appealing to Parkies for several reasons. It can be done alone or in a group, it does not require equipment or a lot of space, and it does not require a special facility. Tai chi exercises your muscles and your mind at the same time. The movements are gentle and slow, which is great for seniors and people who have a great deal of rigidity or balance problems.

Tai chi has been gaining popularity with PD patients in recent years. People with Parkinson's at the Struthers Parkinson's Center in Golden Valley, Minnesota, have had access to tai chi for many years.

A University of Florida–Jacksonville study followed three hundred Parkinson's patients and found that those who attended a weekly tai chi class for twelve weeks were less likely to experience worsening of their symptoms or motor function than those who did not.[5]

Yoga

Yoga was begun in India more than five thousand years ago. It is not a religion, nor is it merely a form of stretching. Yoga is considered to be a philosophy that unites the body, mind, and breath, and focuses them inward. This is supposed to make us more aware of our thoughts and feelings. Practicing yoga does not mean that you need to change your religious beliefs or be able to pull your legs up behind your neck.

There are several different types of yoga, and all involve positioning your body in a pose, or asana. Many of the poses look intimidating, but a good instructor with knowledge of PD will not push you to achieve a position that will hurt you. That is probably the most important criterion in choosing a yoga instructor for us Parkies.

Yoga has been shown to yield many of the same benefits as tai chi, such as improved mood, better balance and flexibility, and a lower stress level.[6]

As with any movement-related activity, be sure to start slowly. Make sure that your surroundings are safe—nothing nearby that's likely to make you trip or fall. Don't try to do yoga when your medication (if you are taking any) is not working. Also, you shouldn't eat for two to three hours prior to yoga, if possible, because you will be twisting your body (gently) and your stomach may rebel.

The best way to begin looking for PD-friendly yoga in your area is to ask your health-care provider. Local health clubs, Ys, and schools may also offer classes.

Coenzyme Q10

Coenzyme Q10 (**CoQ10**), also known as ubiquinone, is an enzyme produced by mitochondrial (energy-producing) cells in our bodies. It is a potent antioxidant, reacting with free radicals before they can cause cell death, and therefore is believed to have at least some neuroprotective qualities.

Research has shown that people who are in the early stages of PD and not yet on any medication have reduced levels of CoQ10 in their bodies. A 2002 study published in the journal *Archives of Neurology* found that the group of these early-stage people with Parkinson's who received doses of 1,200 milligrams of CoQ10 per day deteriorated much less on the UPDRS disability scale (6.7 points versus 12 points for patients receiving no CoQ10). Those patients also had much less decline (44 percent) in their mental function, movement, and activities of daily living.[7] Follow-up studies are being conducted now by the National Institute of Neurological Disorders and Stroke to attempt to replicate the results.

Supplemental CoQ10 in the form of tablets is now available at pharmacies, health food stores, and Internet Web sites. Many people with Parkinson's began taking CoQ10 after the 2002 study and report that they believe the supplement does have beneficial effects.

THINGS TO CONSIDER WHEN TAKING CoQ10

CoQ10 is regulated as a food, not a drug, so there is no federal oversight to ensure quality control. In other words, no one is making sure that you are getting what you pay for. There are two different forms of CoQ10: the TRANS form, which was used in the study, and the CIS form.

If you want to follow the same regimen as people in the study, you will need to take 1,200 mg/day of the TRANS form of the supplement. The study used CoQ10 made by the Vitaline company. A month's supply will cost you around two hundred dollars. There are other suppliers of the supplement, but a survey by ConsumerLab.com found that not all CoQ10 is created equal. The testing firm, which claims to have no financial connection to any of the companies whose products were tested, found that three products out of thirty-two had levels of CoQ10 different from those listed on the label. In fact, one brand did not contain any of the enzyme![8]

Insurance companies do not generally cover nutritional supplements. The CIS form of the supplement is cheaper and more readily available, but that form wasn't studied, so we don't know whether it would yield the same results.

We also do not know whether a higher dose of CoQ10 could produce better results. The doses studied were 300, 600, and 1,200 mg/day, respectively, and only the 1,200 mg/day group showed statistically significant improvement.

Even through our bodies make CoQ10, the nutritional supplement form has been found to interact with blood-thinning medications, such as Warfarin, so be sure to consult your doctor if you decide to try it.

The National Institutes of Health are continuing to study CoQ10 and other substances for their neuroprotective abilities, so check their Web site periodically for updates on their findings.

IN A SENTENCE:

> *Massage, yoga, tai chi, Coenzyme Q10, and other supplements and herbal remedies are all ways you might try to minimize or alleviate some of your PD symptoms.*

learning

Be an Active Participant in Your Care

YOU OWE it to yourself and to your family to get the best care that you can afford. By finding a health-care provider whom you trust, early in your disease, you will be getting the best possible start to your treatment. That starts with a physician who is knowledgeable about PD.

> Be informed about your own medical care. Do research and be proactive about your treatment. Don't blindly accept everything the doctor tells you. I wish I had been told about movement disorder specialists, and the fact that they specialize in PD (and other movement disorders). The general neurologist I went to didn't know that my frozen shoulder was PD-related. —MARCIE, *diagnosed at 37*

Doctors can be ignorant, even rude

A study released in April 2005 found that 90 percent of the members of the Parkinson's Disease Society in the United

Kingdom felt that their physicians do not know enough about PD.[9] Although no similar survey has been done here in the United States, conversations I have had with Americans with PD prove that many share that sentiment.

Sadly, my survey respondents were able to give very specific answers about experiences with uninformed or ill-informed doctors, which indicates to me that they were not making generalizations. In addition to becoming better educated on how to diagnose PD, physicians may also require some training in tact and compassion so that they don't say things so bluntly, as Patrick's neurologist did, who "told me I'd wind up in an old people's home."

> The neuro spent ten minutes yelling at me for having "bad" insurance. Then he wrote a letter to my internist telling her that he thought I had PD. My internist, just like the neuro, never told me I was thought to have PD. She just said, "Come back to me if you start falling down." —LINDA, *who was diagnosed more than eight years ago at age 46*

> I retired early after a twenty-two-year career in law enforcement after three or four years of declining vigor and physical abilities. About a year prior to retiring I asked my family physician why I was shaking and sometimes choking. I asked if it could be Parkinson's. He said no and didn't recommend seeing a neurologist until I confronted him again about a year later. The result of the delay in diagnosis will cost me hundreds of thousands of dollars in disability payments, since I retired early. —MIKE, *diagnosed at 52*

Many of us were raised to believe that physicians are infallible and not to be questioned. I know that I grew up with that unspoken message. The ordeal that I experienced trying to get my PD diagnosed changed all that. My survey results indicate that I was not the only one to have an arduous journey from initial symptoms to likely diagnosis.

Not all doctors are bad apples

While there are definitely some "bad apples" out there practicing medicine, there are many compassionate, trustworthy providers who offer excellent care. Joy, diagnosed at age forty-six, says, "Right after giving me the PD diagnosis, my first neurologist (a woman) told me I should be able to lead a fairly normal life, with the proper medications."

Right now, you're probably saying to yourself: "I have enough to do just coming to terms with having this disease. I never asked to be an amateur pharmacist/social worker/dietician!" That is true for all of us, I would venture to say. But only you can tell if the relationship is working or not, and a good way to determine whether or not your practitioner is the right one for you is to do some research.

Because of PD's varying effects on each person, it is critical for you to be up-front and honest with yourself and your doctor about your symptoms and your treatment. Coming to terms with a new symptom or the worsening of an existing one is difficult enough to deal with on your own, but waiting for your doctor or someone else to notice it before you seek treatment harms only you.

Choosing your health-care provider

In some ways, choosing your health-care provider is like choosing a mate or a business partner. Let's face it—you will most likely be seeing this person for years, and if you don't like him or her, it will not be productive for either one of you. Here are some questions to ask yourself as you evaluate prospective practitioners:

Do I know anyone else who has seen this provider? Getting an opinion from another person with Parkinson's who has seen this doctor can sometimes greatly inform your selection process.

Do I trust this person? If something about the doctor/nurse/practitioner makes you nervous, think about whether you have gotten that feeling from all of the providers you have seen, or just this one.

Does this person seem knowledgeable about Parkinson's disease? Does he keep up on and make use of the latest scientific developments?

How many people with PD has she treated? Ask if any of those people would be willing to contact you to act as a reference.

How does he feel about second opinions? A doctor who says, "None of my patients has ever had to ask for a second opinion," may not be willing to acknowledge mistakes.

Is he or she a neurologist? There is no rule that says you must be treated by a neurologist to get good medical care for your Parkinson's, but neurologists—and more specifically, movement disorder specialists—are most likely to be aware of the latest information on treatment.

Is he a movement disorder specialist? Movement disorder clinics see a large clientele of people with Parkinson's and often have additional resources and complementary therapies to offer.

Should you choose a family doctor, neurologist, or movement disorder specialist?

When most people are diagnosed with PD, it is by their general practitioner or internist—their "family doctor." Chances are that she has not had much training in Parkinson's disease–related issues since medical school, unless you are in an urban area and there happen to be several cases of PD among her patients. That level of care may be perfectly adequate for your treatment.

Many of my Parkie friends were diagnosed by their regular physicians but choose to see a neurologist as their disease progresses. A neurologist is a doctor who has completed a three-year program that deals with brain disorders and diseases. Some of this training is in psychiatry as well as neurology. Neurologists are not required to take a board certification exam in order to practice, but the test they do have to take, like the bar exam for attorneys, does ensure a basic level of competence.

Movement disorder specialists are neurologists who have studied an additional one to three years in a movement disorder program. Movement disorders include diseases such as Parkinson's disease, multiple sclerosis, and ALS. There is no additional board certification for this position, but a physician who has completed such a program will usually have a diploma or certificate displayed in her office.[10]

A number of centers around the country specialize in the treatment of Parkinson's disease and other movement disorders (see Resources). If you live near one of these facilities, you may want to check into receiving treatment from a physician whose specialty is PD. This gives you an even better chance of receiving the best care possible.

Other factors in choosing your physician

There are other issues you should consider when choosing a physician, such as the provider's proximity to your home, whether they accept your insurance coverage, and the cost of treatment. Many people with Parkinson's do choose to pay more or travel farther to see a health-care provider whom they trust and whom they feel is well informed. Appointments with neurologists or movement disorder specialists often take place six months apart, so distance from the provider need not be a big limiting factor, depending on your physical mobility right now.

Let your doctor know that you have questions

Being diagnosed with a chronic illness is a lot to absorb in one doctor's visit. You will undoubtedly have questions that you want answered, and physicians—especially those who work for health-maintenance organizations (HMOs)—have limited time. You can increase the chances of getting your questions answered if you prepare a list ahead of time. Prioritize your questions, and ask the ones about which you are most concerned or interested first in case you run out of time.

You can also let staff know when you are making your appointment that you have some questions for the doctor. If that is not possible, let the nurse know when she is taking your vital signs. If you can get the questions to the doctor before your visit, she may be able to have the answers ready at your appointment. Remember, PD is a complex disease, and you could very easily have questions that your physician cannot answer on the spot.

Some health-care providers are willing to accept, and perhaps even answer, some questions via e-mail. Find out if your doctor is one of them. You are more likely to get a thorough response if the physician has had time to think about or research your question. It can also keep the appointment schedule moving, because your doctor can either plan for a longer visit with you or have information ready when you arrive. If you do not have access to e-mail in your home, check with your children or neighbors to see if they would be willing to help you.

Find someone to advocate for you

Nearly everyone experiences some apprehension about going to the doctor, even if he or she has been your physician for years. That anxiety is compounded when you are seeing someone whom you don't know and because a chronic disease is stressful. In order to make sure that you are able to raise the concerns you have and know that you understand all the components of your treatment plan, it is a good idea to bring someone with you to all of your appointments. That person may be your spouse, your adult child, a friend—someone who will speak up on your behalf if you are not being heard (sometimes literally) and who will collect the prescriptions, referrals, paperwork, and other paraphernalia that seems to go along with most any doctor visit.

I could never have navigated my way through the bureaucracy and confusion of my health plan without the assistance and advocacy of my psychologist at the time, Stan Johnson. In addition to helping me to develop coping mechanisms for dealing with the depression and anxiety I was feeling about not knowing what was wrong, Stan made calls, pushed for referrals, and personally attested to the symptoms he had seen me manifest. Thanks, Stan!

Have someone along to take notes

Another reason to have a companion or advocate with you is to make sure you understand what is being said. Especially now, when you are still adjusting to the news of having PD, your doctor may suggest or prescribe courses of treatment that go right over your head because your mind can't absorb any new information. If you have someone with you who will take notes, it will be much less likely that you will overlook something important.

IN A SENTENCE:

> *Don't be afraid to ask questions and check that you have a doctor whom you can trust—one who knows about the most current treatments and complementary therapies.*

Parkinson's Can Bring Many Gifts

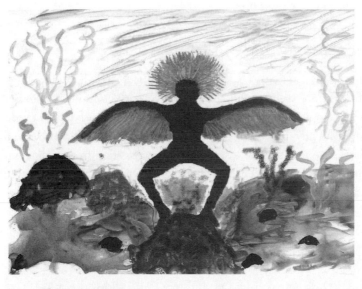

Phoenix Rising
From the ashes of the broken identity that
crashed and burned upon impact of diagnosis
has risen a newborn self,
who is experiencing the world as if for the first time.
She toddles about unsteadily, clutching

seemingly random objects in tight fists,
tasting and touching them for hours as if
suckling nectar for her nascent soul.
She uses the disparate treasures—
words and beads,
music and metal,
paint and paper—
to assemble the alphabet for the
language of her new homeland,
encoding emotions into collages of communication
that she will use to announce her rebirth.

© *Poem and artwork by Jackie Hunt Christensen 2005*

IN THE early years after your diagnosis, you will be able to do everything you did before PD, but you may not be able to do it as fast or as well. There will be some exceptions, but in general, you are not likely to be seriously handicapped by PD in the beginning. If you were putting off perfecting your fly-fishing or quilting or going hiking in Nepal until your "golden years," wait no longer. They are here and now!

Enjoy recreational and outdoor activities

Many recreational activities, such as running, racquetball, hiking, bicycling, and fishing, are still possible, as long as you use common sense. For example, if you enjoy running but have a tendency to trip or fall, you might try a treadmill with grab bars along the sides. If you are a hiker, you may need to allow more time and choose a shorter hike with smoother terrain, but beyond that, you will most likely be able to enjoy that pastime for years to come. And medication can usually help to alleviate many of the symptoms that led to your diagnosis.

Develop new hobbies

Before my PD diagnosis, I had no hobbies. All I did was work. I have developed a number of new hobbies, many of which call for manual dexterity. Sometimes I need to perform them more slowly or ask for help, but I can still enjoy them. Some hobbies—cooking and fishing, for example— are activities that I can do with my family. Here are examples of some of the things I do now that I didn't do before I got Parkinson's disease:

- ○ Write poetry and short stories
- ○ Make beaded jewelry
- ○ Paint with watercolors
- ○ Sketch/draw
- ○ Go fishing

I recall that at one of the first PD support group meetings I attended, we had a guest speaker who came to tell us about his newest hobby: skydiving. I believe he was eighty-one years old! Then there's Gary, from my support group, who is truly an inspiration, especially to those of us who crave excitement. In the five or so years that I have known him, this retired math professor has been to Nepal and China—on his own, has gone ice-climbing and bungee-jumping, and does beautiful woodworking.

Take advantage of new opportunities

Many people believe in the adage, "When God closes a door, he opens a window." You do not have to be a religious person to realize that your perception of a situation will affect your response to it.

Give yourself permission to explore, brainstorm, and think "outside the box." Opportunities have a way of presenting themselves, if you are paying attention. If there are things that you always wanted to do but never had the time, or places you wanted to visit when you retired, consider doing them now, while you know you can enjoy them. That way, you won't look back with regret someday. In seizing the moments now, you may stumble across a new hobby or even a new career.

I am not alone in my discovery of artistic talents after my PD was diagnosed. I know many Parkies who have begun such crafts as woodworking, photography, beadwork, painting, and drawing after the appearance of their disease.

Get involved in your community

For many with PD, this disease presents an opportunity to get involved in their community. That may mean their geographic area or the community of people affected by Parkinson's. My good friend Mike O'Leary of Phoenix is an example of both. Before PD, Mike worked at a local public utility and led a quiet life. He is no longer able to work because of his PD, but he has channeled his energy into helping others with PD to cope with the disease. He makes a point of reaching out to those who are newly diagnosed and is always there with an e-mail, phone call, or even a visit if someone needs emotional support.

Filmmaker Robert Cochrane and his father, Dan, who has PD, combined their shared love of baseball with a desire to educate others about Parkinson's disease. The result: a whirlwind tour of all thirty major league baseball parks in one summer that included fund-raisers and educational sessions for PD awareness at each stop. The Cochranes made a documentary film of their expedition titled *The Boys of Summer*.

Be spontaneous!

Most of the Parkies I know, myself included, like to have everything planned. Well, PD has thrown a monkey wrench into that idea, hasn't it? So why not embrace it! If you are feeling good today, go on a picnic. Go dancing. Take a walk with your sweetheart. None of us knows how long our honeymoon with PD will last, so make the most of it.

There is always someone in worse shape than you are

If you haven't already read *Tuesdays with Morrie: An Old Man, A Young Man, and Life's Greatest Lesson,* by Mitch Albom, I highly recommend buying it or checking it out from the library. Morrie was a man with ALS (also known as Lou Gehrig's disease). Even when he was unable to move, he was cheerful and optimistic. It wasn't that he was ignoring his feelings of anger, sadness, and frustration; he allocated a few minutes of each day to feeling them and then put them aside. He simply did not let them rule his life.

IN A SENTENCE:

> Many people with Parkinson's have responded to their diagnosis by developing a new career, finding hobbies, or getting involved with their community.

learning

Why All Those Warning Labels?

THE STICKERS and labels that come with prescription and over-the-counter medications may seem like a waste of paper at times, but they are very important. Seniors, in particular, need to be sure to inform their doctors and pharmacists about drugs, herbal remedies, and vitamin supplements that they are already taking. There are numerous physical changes that come with age that affect how our bodies metabolize compounds.

If you have other health conditions in addition to Parkinson's disease, be sure that your neurologist or physician managing your PD is aware of this, even if you are not currently taking any medication for that condition. Certain health problems, such as skin cancer, heart disease, or kidney disease, for instance, can be worsened by taking Sinemet.

Read the warnings—heed the warnings

At times, it may seem like all of those stickers on your prescription bottles are rather excessive, but they really are there for a reason. Especially if you are on more than one medication, it's important to look at the labels and any package inserts or additional information that comes with a new prescription so you can familiarize yourself with what medication should do and side effects you could encounter.

Whenever you pick up a refill, be sure to check the label for any new stickers. As new research appears and the Food and Drug Administration (FDA) issues warnings, important new information may be added. Usually if this occurs, your pharmacist will call it to your attention.

Seniors should be especially careful

As we age, our metabolism changes and we need less of a drug to achieve the desired effect. Seniors should take this into consideration. In general, elderly people have more medical problems and thus are likely to be on more than one medication. The more medications, vitamins, minerals, and herbal supplements you take, the higher your risk of drug interactions.

Know what your prescription label means

The label on your prescription bottle gives you a lot of important information. Following, you will see a sample prescription label. It tells you more than just the name of the prescription and who it is for. The refill phone number tells you where to call to get more of the medication. Many refill lines are automated now so that you can call the listed phone number, follow the voice prompts that ask you to punch in the prescription number on your phone key pad and confirm your identity and the location where you're going to pick up the prescription, and you're done. This is handy if you are like me and tend to remember the need for medication refills when the pharmacy is closed.

Keeping track of the number of refills is important, because PD meds and antidepressants must be taken consistently in order to work properly, and you don't want to run out.

The provider listed on the label is the physician who prescribed the medication. When you need additional refills authorized, this is the person whose office you contact to obtain more. (Usually physicians have a nurse who is in charge of handling prescription requests.)

Reading Your Prescription Label

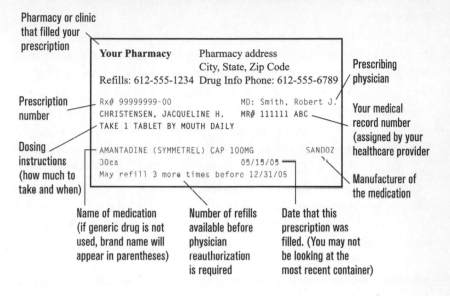

Pharmacy or clinic that filled your prescription

Prescription number

Dosing instructions (how much to take and when)

Prescribing physician

Your medical record number (assigned by your healthcare provider)

Manufacturer of the medication

Name of medication (if generic drug is not used, brand name will appear in parentheses)

Number of refills available before physician reauthorization is required

Date that this prescription was filled. (You may not be looking at the most recent container)

Pay attention to the stickers

The colored stickers found on prescription containers give additional information about dosing (e.g., "Take with Food" or "Do Not Take Antacids While Using This Medication." They can also be used to give important warnings about side effects of the medication (e.g., "This medication may cause dizziness" or "May cause drowsiness. Alcohol may intensify this effect. Use care when operating a car or dangerous machinery.").

Contact your doctor if you don't feel right

This past summer, my antidepressant medication was increased because I just wasn't feeling motivated and wasn't enjoying even my favorite hobbies. The higher medication dose began on a Tuesday. Three days later, when I left my house for a board meeting at a building I'd been to several times before, I found that after driving around for thirty minutes (about fifteen minutes after I *should* have arrived at the building) I was totally lost. I was able to reach a good friend, who helped me to calm down and who also had some sort of Global Positioning System (GPS) software that literally allowed him to "talk me in" to the address I was looking for, as an air-traffic controller might do.

As if that disorienting experience weren't frightening enough, I noticed that when I attended an Eric Clapton concert two nights later, I felt an overwhelming urge to try to fly from my upper-deck seat in the arena. I did not feel suicidal. It was as if I kept seeing a video or movie of myself flying over the crowd like Wonder Woman. Luckily, I knew that this was not a rational thought, so I did not attempt it. But I did spend a very nerve-wracking forty minutes literally holding on to my chair for dear life! I called my neurologist the next day, and his nurse immediately understood the symptoms.

My dose of the medication was modified, and I was able to overcome many of my worst symptoms of depression and get rid of the confusion and the urge to fly. This was a very frightening experience that made me even more aware of the importance of tracking my response to medications.

Those stickers you see on the side of your prescription bottle mean that lab tests or research studies have found that those effects are likely to occur. But their presence on the medication bottle does not mean that you are guaranteed to experience all of those side effects. Keep in mind that since everyone's body chemistry is different, you could also experience side effects that are not listed on the pill bottle because they are more rare.

Keep a medication diary

All of this makes it even more important for you to keep a medication or drug diary. The examples contained in the following table highlight some of the consequences of not being aware of your medications.

If you have questions about your medication, talk to your pharmacist. It is his job to know about drug interactions and side effects, whereas your doctor often just knows what symptoms that drug is supposed to treat.

Potential Drug Interactions

Medication	Taken for	Interacts With	Taken for	Effects
Carbidopa-Levodopa (Sinemet®)	Dopamine precursor/replacement	Lorazepam (Ativan®)	Anxiety	Ativan could reduce effectiveness of Sinemet. A doctor should monitor.
Pramipexole (Mirapex®)	Dopamine agonist	Lorazepam (Ativan)	Anxiety	Both drugs can cause drowsiness, dizziness. Taking both medications can have synergistic effects, especially in elderly or debilitated patients.
Ropinirole (Requip®)	Dopamine agonist	Sleep aids, antihistamines, antipsychotics, antidepressants, alcohol	Sleep, allergies, psychoses, depression	Taking any one of these medications with Requip could make you very drowsy. Consult your doctor before taking any of these products.
Buproprion (Wellbutrin®)	Antidepressant	Vitamins, minerals, OTC medications	Nutritional supplements, cold remedies	May interact with this drug or reduce its effectiveness. Check with your doctor before taking any other medications or products.

Source: Drug Information Online, www.drugs.com (accessed April 28–May 5, 2005).

Sources of drug information

Although it is no substitute for consulting your pharmacist or physician, it can be helpful to have a copy of the *Physician's Desk Reference*, also known as the PDR, the *Consumer Guide to Prescription Drugs*, and the *Merck Manual*. These books allow you to cross-reference your medications at any time. However, if you are on a new medication, it may not always be listed in the edition you have.

You can also keep track of the patient information that comes with your medications by putting them in a binder.

Lastly, there are numerous databases online that allow you to enter all of the medications you take and get a list of interactions, if any. A few of these Web sites also have some information on interaction with herbal supplements.

IN A SENTENCE:

> *Warning labels and stickers on prescriptions should be heeded, especially by the elderly.*

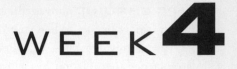

Care Partners Need Love, Too

My Caregiver
They are the ones we count on
To get us through the day.
The dreams they held onto for so long
Are safely packed away.
They care their own burden
And now have ours there too.
Without their help and patience
There's not much we could do.
There must be times they want to flee
To a life which has no cares
But they would never leave us behind
They have made our lifestyle, theirs.
Even though they are not the ones
Whose disease has made them ill
It affects them just as much or more
And for them there is no pill
So I want to take a moment
To tell them how I feel
The love and admiration
For them is very real.
I realize the sacrifice
That they have made for me
There is no one greater in my life
[than] the ones who care for me.

Jeannie Lewis, diagnosed at age 43. Used with permission.

ANY CHRONIC illness affects every family member, even if that impact is not obvious. When your care partner is a spouse or family member, your family dynamics will change. If a friend or neighbor is a primary care partner, that relationship will also change.

Care partners are in a difficult position

Care partners who are also spouses or life partners of someone with PD are in the unenviable position of watching their mate begin to struggle with movements or tasks and walk that fine line between offering assistance out of love and holding back because they know their loved one wants to remain independent as long as possible.

You need to remember that when your partner offers to help you get dressed, cut food, and so on, she almost certainly is doing so out of love for you. She is not trying to make you feel like a child or an invalid. The next time you find yourself about to retort," I can do it myself!" pause a moment to think about why you are resistant to help. Is it because you really could use some assistance but are afraid to admit it? Would there be any harm done (except maybe to your pride) if you said, "Why, yes, actually, I would like some help?"

Care partner versus caregiver

Many of the Parkies I know have expressed a strong dislike for the term "caregiver," because they think it implies that the relationship is very one-sided. While it is true that you may reach a point in your relationship with your partner where he or she is doing most of the giving, it doesn't have to be that way. Especially now, early in your disease, you have plenty to offer your care partner.

I recommend having a conversation with your partner about the division of labor in your relationship. That may refer to concrete tasks like housework or bookkeeping, or it may refer to emotional support. Perhaps your spouse would like you to just listen to him talk about his day at work or with the grandchildren for thirty minutes when he gets home. I am sure that if you try, you will be able to come up with a plan in which you can continue to be care partners to each other.

Care partners: take time for yourself!

As a care partner, taking time for yourself is critical for your own health and well-being as well as for your relationship with the person with PD! If you do not make time to do things that are not PD-related, you will be under much more stress, which can cause depression and anxiety, and you may become bitter and resentful toward the person with PD.

Family care partners who provide care thirty-six or more hours per week are more likely than non-caregivers to experience symptoms of depression or anxiety. For spouses, the rate is six times higher; for those caring for a parent, the rate is twice as high.[1] So get out there and blow off some steam! It will do everyone involved a world of good.

Being a care partner isn't easy

Being a care partner is not an easy job. Not only can it be physically taxing, but it can also exact a serious psychological toll. Care partners often find themselves battling feelings of stress and isolation, and sometimes this can lead to a change in how they feel about their partner on the whole. I don't think that these feelings are inevitable, but I do think that preventing them takes a lot of work on the part of both the care partner and the person with Parkinson's.

One anonymous care partner who replied to my survey, whose husband was diagnosed at age sixty-seven, wrote:

> The stresses and disappointments of coping with his condition and the limitations it places on his life and mine have eroded my feelings for him. I don't feel like I have a husband—I have a patient. I have learned from this experience that I was not cut out to be a nurse. I enjoy our support group meetings but they are only once a month. We don't see any of the members at other times, although I guess we could. I feel very alone and isolated. I think about asking friends (whom we see only occasionally) for help but I feel they are all very busy with their own lives.

I can attest to the difficulties involved in the caregiver/patient relationship. The physical and cognitive changes that I am experiencing are also affecting my husband. For example, I get frustrated when I cannot zip my jacket. Paul gets frustrated watching me try to zip my jacket, knowing that if he offers to help, I will most likely respond like a petulant two-year-old: "I can do it myself!"

We can't always talk about it in the heat of the moment, but after either of us has had an outburst of frustration, we try to talk about it. Very often, it is the tone of voice in which he offers help or the words he choose, rather than his desire to help, that ticks me off. Likewise, I may respond harshly because I am frustrated with myself, and he may interpret my response as anger directed at him.

Stay in touch with non-PD friends

This may be difficult, but care partners really need to have contact with the outside world. It is very easy to get trapped in the role of "Sheila's care partner" or "Jeff's care partner" and have that serve as your entire identity. It is not realistic or healthy to rely on one person to meet all of your needs. This is true even when we are healthy. You do not love your care partner any less by spending time with friends and confiding in others. Indeed, you are showing that you care about your partner's well-being and that you do not expect him to develop skills that he does not have.

Schedule play dates

Sit down with your care partner and work out some time where she can go off and do as she pleases. Ideally, it would be at least once per week for a few hours. Whenever the weather cooperates, my husband, Paul, goes windsurfing or snowboarding. Sometimes he just putters around in the garage. It is his choice. If I am traveling, as I still often do for PD- or environmental health–related activities, I get a friend or relative to take the kids off his hands. If I am home, we both agree that if I need help with something, I have any number of neighbors, relatives, and friends I will call first so that he can have his time off.

Since I am no longer working outside the home, we have changed our routine of alternating cooking nights. Now I cook nearly every night, and our sons are supposed to deal with the dishes. It's not a perfect system, but one of our goals is to give Paul some downtime when he gets home from work.

A number of resources and support organizations are available to care partners. See Resources for a partial list of contacts that care partners may find useful.

IN A SENTENCE:

> *Care partners need to maintain their physical and mental health for their own well-being as well as yours.*

learning

Utilizing Local Support Services for Physical and Occupational Therapy

MANY PEOPLE think of physical therapy as something that only injured athletes or paraplegics need. In reality, physical therapy can be very beneficial for treating Parkinson's disease–related conditions such as "frozen shoulder," neck and back pain, and walking difficulties that are common in people who are newly diagnosed. In addition, physical therapists (PTs) can provide stretching and strengthening exercises to keep such pain from recurring or at least keep it under control. They may have exercise/movement classes especially for PD patients.

Physical therapy

Physical therapy can help a number of your symptoms. A physical therapist will show you exercises that can help you improve your walk, get you to stand up straighter, make you stronger, and increase your range of motion and flexibility. Depending on your insurance, you'll probably need to be referred by your doctor or have a prescription written to allow you to see a physical therapist.

A physical therapist will give you two different types of exercises or movements to perform. The first type is called *active movement*, or moves that you initiate. The other is called *passive movement*, or those movements that are made by the therapist for you. For example, the therapist might gently turn your head from side to side while supporting your neck. For these movements, your job is to relax as much as possible and let the therapist move your body.

A PT will often give you exercises to do on your own time as well as oversee exercises during your visits. She may prescribe the use of ice packs, heat, electrical stimulation, water therapy, or a combination of all of the above to help ease your symptoms. You may need to go to a clinic to receive some of these treatments, but many can be implemented in your own home.

PTs are also a great resource because they can offer advice on mobility-related equipment, such as canes and walkers, in addition to exercise gear. They will have models for you to "test-drive" and will take measurements and do various tests to make sure that you get the equipment that is right for you. They will see to it that you know how to use it properly, too.

Visits to a PT usually last for a few weeks or months, by which time you will have learned how to maintain your strength and flexibility and have an array of exercises at your disposal to keep you in shape. You can always ask your health-care provider for another referral if you need more visits.

I can't emphasize enough the benefits that I have experienced since I began seeing a PT again. In just a few weeks, I was able to increase the range of motion in my neck and shoulders, and I have much less pain.

Occupational therapy

Occupational therapists (OTs) help people develop new skills in order to adjust their "activities of daily living" (ADLs) to cope with a disease or injury. OTs have gone through considerable training, which enables them to evaluate the way that PD is affecting you and make recommendations for ways you can safely go about your day.

OTs WILL EVALUATE YOUR CAPABILITIES

If you visit an OT, he will observe you going through the motions of tasks that you do every day: brushing your teeth, eating, getting dressed, and so on. He will make a note of tasks that are giving you trouble, and then, if necessary, suggest different ways you can do them more safely. He may also recommend you invest in some adaptive equipment, which are tools that have been modified to help you perform specific actions you have difficulty doing.

OTs WILL CHECK YOUR HOME FOR SAFETY

Oftentimes occupational and physical therapists will work as a team to do an evaluation of your home. The PT may have suggestions or raise issues about your mobility in and around your living space. The OT will be looking for potential hazards, such as stairs that are very steep or do not have railings on both sides; cords, rugs, or door thresholds that could cause you to trip; and so on. He will also want to see you performing tasks that you do at home on a regular basis, such as cooking, cleaning, and working at a computer. At the end of the evaluation, you will get a list of problems that pose an imminent threat to your safety or well-being, a list of issues to monitor, and a list of things that may become an issue at some point in the future.

If you are still working, your OT may want to make a site visit to your workplace. If so, he will offer ideas on how to change your work environment or your work habits so that you can work safely for as long as possible. Some of the changes may be ones that your employer is obligated to make, under the Americans with Disabilities Act (ADA). (More on ADA in Month 10.) Others may merely be suggestions you can try if you are so inclined.

Although working with an OT may sound frightening or daunting, I have found it to be very valuable. I know that my husband was glad to hear someone else warning me about safety issues after he had voiced concern and been ignored. Sometimes it is easier to hear tough suggestions, like "Maybe you should have your driving evaluated," from a disinterested party.

IN A SENTENCE:

> *Physical therapists can give you specific advice on exercises and stretching techniques, and frequently work in tandem with occupational therapists, who can recommend changes to make your home and work environment safer for you.*

FIRST-MONTH MILESTONE

I know it has been a rough month, but you have learned some essential information that will help you to cope on your journey with Parkinson's disease:

○ You have learned about the vast array of physical and mental symptoms that may be affecting you now, or may do so in the future.

○ You have read about and seen some of the gifts that Parkinson's can bring to the lives of others with this disease.

○ You know how to identify people and organizations that can help you and your family with all aspects of PD.

○ You know that it is important for both you and your care partner to learn to delegate some responsibilities and to have a life outside of Parkinson's disease.

The Importance of Support Groups

NO MATTER how strong you are emotionally or physically, coping with PD alone is not a good idea. Humans are social animals, even when we're shaky or stiff. Being in a support group is good for you for a number of reasons:

- ○ It gives you an excuse to get out of the house.
- ○ You will be with people who are more likely than anyone else to understand how you feel.
- ○ You can learn more about the disease and how you might be affected.

Support groups can serve more than one purpose. Some groups, for example, are primarily social. They provide a reason to get out of the house and be around other Parkies. Other groups use a facilitator to moderate or manage the discussion, and serve as a forum to discuss feelings, air frustrations, and ask for feedback or suggestions from other group members.

Attending a support group is not a requirement of PD treatment, and it is okay to wait until you feel like you need one. My goal is to make you aware of the benefits of support groups and ensure that you know how to find one when you need it.

How to find a group

Many hospitals and neurology clinics have support groups. Your doctor may be able to provide you with a list. The American Parkinson's Disease Association (APDA), the National Parkinson Foundation (NPF), and the Parkinson's Disease Foundation (PDF) all have support groups around the country. (See Resources for contact information for each of these organizations.)

There are different types of groups

Some groups are just for people with Parkinson's disease. Others are for people with Parkinson's and their care partners. Many groups bring in guest speakers for some sessions, while some have made the decision to focus solely on providing personal moral support. Look for a group that seems best suited to your needs.

The young-onset PD support group that my husband and I attend is made up of ten or so couples and two or three individuals with PD. We meet once a month for about two and a half hours. At the beginning of each session, we all get together for a brief "check-in," during which each gives an update on how he has been doing since the last meeting. Then we split into two groups: Parkies and care partners. If we have eight or more in each group, we may break into smaller groups to make sure that everyone has a chance to talk.

Before you attend your first meeting

Going to your first meeting can be a terrifying experience, particularly if you have never been in any sort of support group before. In advance of going, I urge you to think about how you typically respond to change or crisis in your life. If you are a person who deals best with incremental change, you might try to find a group that has people who are all newly diagnosed or near your age. If you prefer to know the gamut of possibilities you might be facing or if you don't shock easily, the age range or stage of PD may not make as much difference. Another way to minimize the shock as well as to find the group that best suits your needs is to ask some questions about the group before you go, such as:

○ What is the age range of the attendees?
○ How long has the group been meeting?
○ Does the group have a facilitator? (If so, talking with her ahead of time would be helpful.)
○ Does the group have members in various stages of PD? Are the majority in one stage, and if so, which one?

Unless the group you will be visiting is only for newly diagnosed people, there will probably be at least one person in a more advanced stage of the disease. This experience may scare some people away because they are not ready to face people who are "like that." In other words, they are unprepared to see me wiggling like a human Slinky, or to see a woman whose hands have such rapid violent tremors that you think she might be able to hover above the ground. A man who shuffles and speaks only in a whisper, with no apparent expression, might not seem very welcoming. We all have PD, and it has affected us all differently. Yet we can still confide in one another about our fears of rejection and embarrassment and learn coping strategies from others whose disease is more advanced than our own.

Starting your own group

Perhaps you live in an area where there is not currently a support group. Or maybe there is a group, but it is comprised solely of people in advanced stages of the disease and you are justifiably interested in being with other newly diagnosed people.

Because of privacy rules under the Health Insurance Portability and Accountability Act (HIPAA), usually referred to as "HIP uh," your doctor cannot give you a list of names of other newly diagnosed people. However, if you give your permission, your health-care provider can give your name to other patients as she sees them in appointments.

You may be thinking, "Good grief! I've just been diagnosed with Parkinson's, and now she wants me to start my own support group, too?!" Having been a support group facilitator, I am very aware of how much work it can be to recruit members and build a core group. However, I have also experienced firsthand the benefits of having others in similar circumstances with whom I can discuss what is happening in my life. You may find that having something else on which to focus your energies relieves some of your stress about having Parkinson's disease.

APDA, NPF, and PDF have excellent manuals and resources for support group leaders. Depending upon your location, they may also provide facilitator-training workshops to help you get started.

IN A SENTENCE:

> Support groups are an invaluable way to learn more about Parkinson's disease, get out of your house, and most important, find others who share circumstances similar to yours.

learning

Finding Your Support System

THE USE of the word "system" here is very intentional. As I mentioned in the section on care partners, it is presumptuous and unrealistic to expect one person to be able to meet all of the care needs that will arise as your disease progresses. By now, you have learned a great deal about what the future may hold for you physically and mentally. You have identified potential sources of support: your doctor, physical therapist, occupational therapist, and support group, to name a few.

Plan ahead

It is hard to think about getting help when you don't need it. We tend to be very vague and disorganized. I may tell myself, "If something were to happen to Paul so that he couldn't help me around the house, I am sure I would figure out something." But it's an important part of planning ahead for your future with PD. What would you do if your spouse slipped and broke an ankle and is temporarily immobilized, leaving you to care for the both of you? And of course, we know that at any time, an illness or accident could take our care partner away permanently.

There are many ways to go about identifying who is in your support system and to discover the "holes" in that support network.

One of the biggest hurdles for many of us—I know it is one I keep tripping over—is surrendering my pride and summoning the courage to ask for help, or even to ask for potential help.

Many people find it helpful to actually map out or make a list of people in their support network, specifying who is the contact or responsible party for each particular task or service. For example, I know that I have two particular friends I can contact during the weekdays when I am home alone and just want someone to talk to. Since one is in Washington State and the other is in Michigan, I know that I have to have other people in mind if I need a ride to a doctor's appointment or if I need help with something around the house.

Learn to delegate

You (and your care partner) have some choices to make. How do you want to spend the time that you have now, while you can still do most things that you enjoy without PD interfering too much? Do you want to wallow in self-pity for a while? I needed to do that when I was first diagnosed, and I still retreat to the "pity bog" every now and then. When I decide that I have had enough of the self-pity mud bath, I realize that I could (a) try to pull myself out, with poor odds that I could do it on my own and not without certain exhaustion and possible injury; (b) hope and pray that someone will notice me and offer to rescue me; (c) accept the offer of a helping hand; or (d) call out to a loved one or a friend whom I know well. Although I often hope for a dramatic rescue, I usually make a phone call to someone whom I know will listen to me whine and cry for a while and then help me to develop a plan of action. I would say that at least half the battle of setting up a support system is being willing to relinquish control (or at least the appearance of it) over some of your activities or chores.

Once you have conceded that you could, in some hypothetical situation, allow some other person to attempt to fill your shoes, you need to decide which tasks you are going to release from your grasp.

Let someone else do it

Yes, it is true that no one else can fold the bath towels exactly the way you do, or trim the hedges just so, or use your filing system as quickly and efficiently. But unfortunately, you will reach a point where you will not be able to do it either.

First, you must ask yourself, "Is what I am upset about really worth it?" Is the activity or chore a need, or is it an added bonus? If it is a bonus or luxury, I personally might choose to give it up altogether, rather than have someone else do it, because I am so doggone stubborn. If it is a necessity, then I have another decision to make.

"Do I enjoy this activity or task?" If not, let someone else do it! I look at the situation as God or the Universe or any higher power telling me, "Jackie, I know you hate housework and you aren't very good at it anyway, so take this chance to find someone who truly likes to vacuum. This is your chance to go work on that painting you've wanted to do."

So ask yourself: "Does it have to happen? Does it have to be done by me? Would I allow someone to help me? Does it really need to be done under these time constraints?"

If you are someone like me who prefers to have control (or at least the delusion—I mean, illusion, of it) over what happens in your life, look at it this way: you can create the support system you need with the people you have chosen and with your parameters if you do it now. If you put it off, you may up in a situation where you are not in control, and we don't like that very much, do we?

If you are not like me, think of this time as a second chance at some of the best aspects of childhood. You can get someone else to wash your clothes or clean your room.

Putting together your support team

There are many potential types of support that you may need, so once you have identified them, it is time to begin assembling a team.

INCLUDE YOUR CARE PARTNER

Sit down with your care partner, because this team will be supporting both of you. Discuss which tasks you feel comfortable farming out. Also identify things that need to happen but are "orphans," meaning that no one in your immediate circle knows how to do them. Make a list of needs.

MAKE YOUR LIST OF "DRAFT PICKS"

Identify people whom you like and trust, and ask them to be on the team. Don't just add their name to the list and assume that if a time comes when they are needed, they will be there.

CALL A PRACTICE SESSION

If possible, have a meeting of all team members. If a face-to-face gathering is not possible, try to get everyone on a conference call. As part of this gathering, talk about your hopes and expectations as well as theirs.

Once you have shown them the list of potential tasks, step aside and let your team develop. Allow them to do what they do best, whenever possible. For instance, if your cousin Shanita is a whiz at paperwork management, don't ask her to walk the dog for you.

PASS OUT A TEAM ROSTER

Pick a team "captain." There must be someone who can give direction or instructions to the rest of the team if you are unable to do so.

Make sure that everyone knows who the captain is and how to reach him, and how to reach one another. Make sure your doctor and any other members of your health-care team have a copy as well.

CHEER FROM THE SIDELINES

Let team members do what you have asked them to do, and always remember to express your gratitude.

If you live alone

If you live alone or do not have a large group of family members or nearby friends upon whom you can rely, there are community resources that may be able to help.

If you are on Medicare or public assistance, you have most likely been assigned a case manager or social worker. Her job is to serve as a liaison between you and the government agencies that provide services for people with health problems and disabilities. She should be able to help you to set up your network and identify members.

If not, First Call for Help is a good starting point to help you to identify local resources. Look in the front of your phone book for a section called Community/Human Resources. There will most likely be listings for hotlines run by various organizations that should be able to help you build your team.

Many churches and synagogues routinely "adopt" or "sponsor" people in the community who are in need of assistance. In many cases, you do not need to belong to the congregation or even to be affiliated with that denomination to qualify.

Anita's situation

MY FRIEND Anita lives alone, with no family nearby. As her PD has progressed rapidly over the past year, she has put together a team of people that includes paid personal-care attendants (PCAs), neighbors, friends, and members of our support group. This team is responsible for meeting a variety of her needs, from companionship to physical assistance with personal care to running errands.

While Anita's team is currently meeting many of her needs, I predict that a couple of things will need to change if she is to receive adequate support. Anita is running her team right now, which is very stressful. She will need to find someone to serve as team captain and allow the person to function in that capacity; and additional team members who do not have PD should be recruited. Many of us from the support group don't mind serving on the team, but we have our own health and other issues that may prevent us from being there when we are needed.

Whether you have a care partner or live alone, dealing with your Parkinson's disease does not have to be done alone. There are many options that you can investigate now, before you need them.

IN A SENTENCE:

There are many ways to find support for dealing with your PD, ranging from a network of family and friends, to an organized support group, to an in-person or online loosely knit relationship among a few people with Parkinson's.

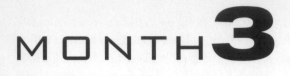

MONTH **3**

living

Useful Assistive Devices for Your Home and Workplace

"BETTER LIVING through gadgets" might become your watchwords as your Parkinson's disease progresses, but better that than "Pride goeth before the fall." Resisting aids, such as canes, walkers, tub-transfer benches, and ramps, because you want to wait until you need them can lead to debilitating falls and broken bones.

PTs and OTs can identify assistive devices and adaptive equipment

Physical therapists (PTs) and occupational therapists (OTs) can help you to assess whether or not you need any assistive devices. I encourage you to schedule a home visit with an OT, a PT, or both. (See Week 4 for more information on physical and occupational therapists.) Your insurance may even cover the evaluation, because the advice PTs and OTs will give you is designed to prevent injury, which saves money for the insurer.

In addition to recommending gadgets to help you or your care partner deal with some aspect of your Parkinson's, an OT may suggest structural changes to your home or apartment. This could include widening your doorways now, if you are doing a remodeling project anyway, or adding a ramp. My husband has expressed concern about a ramp affecting the resale value of our home, but I believe that as the American population ages, such architectural features will increase the value and appeal of a home. Also, ramps can be built so that they can be easily detached.

Medication managers

If you are taking any medication at all, whether it is PD-related or not, medication managers are important. It is very easy—and common—to forget whether you have taken your medication. Having a pillbox with the number of compartments you need can prevent "off" times or overdoses. This is invaluable if you take medication more than once a day or if you take more than one medication. I have found that it is easiest for me to fill the pillbox in the morning when I first get up. Others do it at night before going to sleep. You may need to adapt a pillbox to your schedule. For example, if you take an antidepressant when you get up and before you go to bed, but also take Sinemet before breakfast, lunch, and dinner, you may not be able to find a pillbox with five slots. Get a one-week box and just use five compartments.

A medication reminder or timer is another very useful item. It can help you avoid having your medication wear off before you remember to take the next dose. A vast array of timers are available; many come with a pillbox. Some have loud alarms or a vibrating feature, which is useful if you are hard of hearing or deaf. Large-print or talking alarms are available for those who are visually impaired or blind. There are watches, pendants, key chains, pager-style timers—almost every style you can think of, so there's really no reason not to have one unless you don't take any medication.

Another handy gadget to have is a pill cutter. A pill cutter is a small, inexpensive box with a vertical razor blade that enables you to cut up your pills if or when your doctor tells you to "fractionate" doses of your medication; that is, to take smaller amounts more frequently. These cutters are inexpensive and much more precise than using your teeth! You can use them to cut scored tablets (the kind with a line down the middle) into halves or quarters very easily. Note: Do not use on capsules; and do not use on controlled-release (CR) or sustained-release (SR) types of medication unless your physician tells you to do so.

Dressing aids

There will be times when you feel like buttons and zippers are inventions of Satan, for all the trouble they will give you. Over time, you will probably make changes in your wardrobe to eliminate most of the vexing garments. In the meantime, or for special occasions, you might want to get a button-hook to help you with dress shirts and blouses.

There is also a dressing tool available that's a combination of a long-handled shoehorn and an S-shaped hook that can help you to reach behind you to catch a shirt or sweater sleeve, to get your arm into it.

Home safety

Grab bars for your toilet and bathtub can be very helpful—or very dangerous, if not properly installed. An occupational therapist can evaluate your bathroom and give you tips as to which type to obtain and where to put them.

Consider removing wall-mounted towel bars if you have them above your tub. If you slip, or are turning around in the shower, you could have painful encounters with those bars!

Speaking of slipping, it's also a good idea to invest in a nonskid bath mat or nonskid strips for the floor of your bathtub and shower.

Another helpful safety item is the tub-transfer bench, which allows you to shower while seated. That way, you don't risk getting dizzy as you turn around under the shower. To safely exit the shower, remain seated but swinging your legs around outside the tub. Put both feet on the floor and then stand up slowly. Doing it this way eliminates the "flamingo posture" that many people use—standing with one foot on the wet tub or shower floor while swinging the other over the side. Exiting a tub one leg at a time can result in a nasty fall.

Mobility devices

Many of us view canes or walkers as signs of old age, of surrendering our independence. On the contrary, these devices are intended to help us retain our mobility and independence.

A physical therapist can fit you for a cane and or walker. Don't just go out and buy one for yourself—it's important to get one of the right height so that you will maintain good posture while using it.

Walkers are now available in many styles and even colors! I have a four-wheeled fold-up model with a built-in seat and a detachable wire basket. I have named her Lily Belle, and she always comes with me for airline travel. I can put my computer bag in the wire basket instead of having to carry it. With Lily Belle, I know that I will always have a seat, no matter how congested the gate area may be. I can "gate-check" the walker, which means that the gate agent will put a baggage tag on it. I can use it to walk down the jetway to the plane, and leave it right outside the plane (where strollers and wheelchairs are also left). Airport staff will load it onto the plane and then have it waiting for me when I get off at my destination.

If you are worried that a walker or cane will negatively affect your image or others' perception of you, you can decorate or embellish the item. Make it uniquely yours with paint, decals, ribbons, and so on.

Safety device resources

Goodwill–Easter Seals has lending programs for all kinds of durable medical supplies. canes, walkers, tub-transfer benches, over-the-toilet commodes, grab bars, and many other items. This program allows you to borrow a piece of equipment for up to six months, which gives you time to see if it is helpful, determine whether insurance or Medicare will cover it, and figure out where to purchase one.

Estate sales, rummage sales, and thrift stores can be good inexpensive sources of walkers and tub-transfer benches.

Voice-recognition software

Have you ever wished that instead of having to type out your thoughts on a keyboard, you could just speak and the words would magically appear?

Voice-recognition software is designed to do just that. The technology is not quite perfect, but if you use a computer a lot for work or for writing, this software can be a godsend. You "train" the software after you install it, and then the more you use it, the more accurate the transcription becomes. Two common brands are Dragon "Naturally Speaking" and Via Voice. They are relatively inexpensive, easy to use, and come in basic and professional editions. You can find them at major electronics or office supply stores.

These are just some of the devices that can make life easier for you and your care partner, and help you to maintain your independence for as long as possible.

IN A SENTENCE:

> *Tub-transfer benches, voice-recognition software, canes, walkers, ramps . . . any number of assistive devices can protect you from injury while making life easier.*

learning

Dealing with PD's Possible Effects on Your Voice

PERHAPS YOU, like many of us with PD, did not realize that Parkinson's can affect your speech in many ways. It can be a very early symptom, and it can be a very isolating one. Fortunately, there are things you can do to help with this problem.

Changes in your voice

From childhood through early adulthood, I had a voice that could carry a long way. Sometimes a little too far. It came in handy for raising chants at rallies and marches, speaking to groups of school children about the importance of bearing witness to injustice in the world, and for screaming at the television while watching the Minnesota Vikings take on other teams in the NFL's "black-and-blue" division. Thus, I was surprised that in my early thirties I was being asked to repeat things that I had just said. I would feel very angry, thinking, "Why can't you people just LISTEN to me!" Even after I was diagnosed with PD, I did not know that the volume of my voice could change. I had always associated a quavering, tremulous voice, like Katharine Hepburn's, with PD. (Actually, though, Katharine Hepburn had essential tremor, not Parkinson's disease.)

It was only when my movement disorder specialist asked if I had noticed any changes in my voice or whether I was being asked to repeat things that I expressed this frustration. Dr. Tuite explained that PD can affect the sound level of your voice, your ability to pronounce words clearly, and your vocal expression without your being aware that this is happening.

Voice/speech therapy can be extremely helpful

Dr. Tuite referred me to a speech therapist, who gave me a variety of tests that included saying tongue-twisters, repeating certain words, singing musical scales, and reading aloud. Most of these exercises were recorded and played back to me, and I remember being astounded that many of the sentences or sounds that I had felt I had practically screamed were actually normal to low volume. This has been a big adjustment and one with which I still struggle. I am accustomed to being told, "Shut up!" rather than, "Speak up!"

I never thought that singing along with the radio in my car would be part of my therapy, but it felt great to have that embarrassing pastime validated! (I am not so sure that my husband and sons are thrilled.) Some of the other exercises and tips given by my speech therapist include:

❍ Breathe! You need adequate air in your lungs to project your voice.
❍ Speak slowly. Otherwise, your speech may sound slurred or garbled.
❍ Think "loud." Imagine yourself speaking in a loud, strong voice and you will.
❍ Read aloud. This is also a great way to spend quality time with your spouse, child, or grandchild. If you have no one in your home with whom you can practice, try volunteering at a library, senior center, school, or church. Reading aloud will help your speech volume, your pronunciation, and your vocal expression.
❍ Give your listeners permission to let you know when they cannot hear you. They do not necessarily even need to say, "I can't hear you." If it makes you feel better, ask them to use a sign, such as raising their hand or cupping one hand around an ear.
❍ Make eye contact. Look at the people to whom you are speaking. If you have your back turned to them, it will make it even more difficult for them to hear you.

Changes in your speech can affect your relationships

Popular culture often perpetuates the stereotype that men and women—especially husbands and wives—don't listen to each other. It has been a real struggle in my household at times, because I will be absolutely positive that I have asked my husband or one of my kids to do something—answer the phone, feed the dog, close the door—and my request is not fulfilled. Instead of immediately going ballistic and saying, "#*@&^! I thought I told you to _____!" I need to be certain that I have said my request loudly enough that they actually could have heard it. This often means repeating what I have said. I have explicitly given permission to my husband, sons, other family members, and friends to tell me if they cannot hear me.

If you find yourself feeling slighted—"Why did that store clerk take his order first? Didn't she hear me say I was next?" "Hey! I called 'Bingo' before she did"—ask people you trust (your spouse, children, pastor, close friends) to give you their honest opinion as to whether you are often hard to hear.

While you are asking for feedback, ask your loved ones to tell you if your voice sounds emotionless or flat. Parkinson's also affects the tone of your voice, which conveys how you feel. People who are unaware of this symptom of PD may interpret your lack of inflection as a sign of boredom, anger, or self-importance.

Parkinson's disease can make speaking more difficult at a time when talking with your loved ones and friends is more important than ever. For me, the way that PD affects my voice, taking away the inflection and the rhythm of my speech, has been one of the most difficult symptoms for me. I am shy around people I don't know, but when I am with friends and loved ones, I like to talk a lot. Mercifully, this condition is most pronounced only when I am "off," or if I am very stressed out.

Occasions of stress are when you are most likely to need help, but you have to overcome pride as well as speech that is slow, soft, and without expression. People who are unfamiliar with PD or whom you don't see very often may need to be reminded about how PD may affect your voice. Otherwise, you may be misunderstood, such as when an urgent or annoying situation is not taken seriously because you don't sound upset.

Lee Silverman Voice Treatment

THIS WIDELY acclaimed therapeutic approach "centers on a very specific therapeutic target: increased vocal loudness. This key target acts as a 'trigger' to increase effort and coordination across the speech production system."[1] LSVT has more than fifteen years' and $5 million worth of studies to support its claims about being the most effective voice treatment for people with PD.

MIKE'S EXPERIENCE WITH LSVT

I realized early that my voice was getting low, but I was too stubborn to admit it. What was the clue? Almost everybody I talked to asked me to repeat myself, and my stubbornness didn't allow me to see the obvious.

I met Dr. Cynthia Fox from the University of Arizona and executive vice president of the LSVT Foundation at the 2004 Parkinson's Action Network (PAN) forum. I sat through one of her talks on the voice therapy, and although it sounded like it made sense, I still did not put two and two together.

Not long after the forum, Dr. Fox contacted me to see if I would participate in a case study she was doing in collaboration with UCSF [University of California at San Francisco] to see the effects of LSVT on the brain. I was sent to San Francisco to have my brain imaged by an MEG machine [Magnetoencephalography, which scans for spontaneous magnetic brain activity that is generated by neurons in the brain], then to the University of Arizona for four weeks of voice therapy, then back to San Francisco for another brain imaging. The results of the imaging went to Rome with Dr. Fox to present to the World Movement Disorder Conference. For me, it was an eye-opener. Dr. Fox had recorded me reading the same passage at the beginning of the course, after two weeks, and at the end. What an amazing difference. I still have that tape and do listen to it once in a while, to remind myself to THINK LOUD!! The only real problem is that the test subject didn't get to Rome with the presentation!

You can learn more about the Lee Silverman Voice Treatment (LSVT) program by visiting www.lsvt.org/main_site.htm/.

Come up with a signal

Use "marital Morse code"—a series of winks or blinks or some type of signal to your partner that can mean, "Hey, I could use some help here!" or "I'm doing fine." These little tricks can prevent major relationship warfare in public places. My in-laws, neither of whom has PD, have a clever way of letting each other know if too much free advice is being offered. One will say, "Who is doing this?" which means "I am doing this and if I want your input, I will ask for it, thankyouverymuch."

Find a speech therapist

Look for a therapist who is accustomed to dealing with Parkinson's patients. If your doctor does not know any speech therapists, or if you have trouble finding one in your area, consult Resources for the list of Udall Centers or National Parkinson Foundation Centers of Excellence. They may know someone in your area or may be able to provide you with the service at their own nearby location. Another idea is to check out clinical/research trials for speech therapy opportunities. You still have a lot to say. Make sure that others hear it by getting speech therapy if you need it.

IN A SENTENCE:

> *Voice therapy can help you cope with the loss of volume and inflection that can come with PD.*

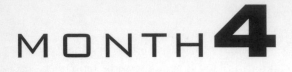

MONTH 4

living

Give Your Care Partner a Break

IF WE are lucky enough to have a care partner in our lives, in most cases that individual is a spouse or partner. Parkinson's disease can change the dynamic of long-term love relationships. Even though many of us included the phrase "in sickness and in health" in our marriage vows or commitment ceremonies, I think that few actually thought about what "sickness" could mean.

Avoiding burnout

We want to have our care partners with us for the long haul. Indeed, the longer we have the disease, the more we will need them to be present. So it is important for us to help our care partners avoid burnout.

Our loved ones may be completely unaware of how overwhelmed they are feeling. There are a number of physical and mental symptoms that can help you both to assess whether your care partner is reaching his or her limit.

Burnout Warning Signs

PHYSICAL SYMPTOMS	EMOTIONAL SYMPTOMS
Headaches	Depression
Digestive problems	Increased anger
Sleep deprivation	Emotional exhaustion
Heartburn	Fatigue
Chronic back pain	Increased anxiety
Other muscle tensions	Preoccupation with death and
Loss of appetite	dying
Weight gain	Low self-esteem
	Apathy
	Increased use of nicotine/
	alcohol/drugs
	Isolation
	Withdrawal
	Memory loss

Reprinted from Neufeld, "Coping with Caregiver Burnout."

If you suspect burnout, I recommend making a list of the signs that you believe your care partner has exhibited and concrete examples. You are not building a criminal case, so there is no need to list every instance of a symptom or behavior. However, your loved one is more likely to acknowledge the situation if you can give him some specifics.

Depending upon your care partner's personality, it may be useful to discuss the issue directly. Choose a quiet moment when the two of you are alone and say something like, "Honey, I'm worried about you. It seems like you are having a lot of headaches, and you're always tired. You don't see much of your friends these days. Maybe you need a night out?" Then you can talk about how to make that happen.

If your loved one is the stoic type who will not admit to feeling overwhelmed, you can try to orchestrate some time off without saying, "It's for your own good."

I have used both approaches with Paul. Sometimes I tell him to go windsurfing or go out with a friend after work. We both work at telling each other if we think one of us is overworked. And on occasion, I will organize an outing or trip for him. (One of my well-meaning but poorly planned efforts will go down in family history. Last year, right before Christmas, I noticed that Paul seemed to be at the end of his rope, so I decided he needed a vacation. He had mentioned on more than one occasion that he would like to try windsurfing at South Padre Island, Texas. I did some searching on the Internet and discovered that I had enough frequent flyer miles on one of the airlines to get him to Corpus Christi over Christmas. I booked him a rental car and a hotel room on the beach. It wasn't until he called me at 2:00 a.m.—more than three hours after I'd expected to hear from him—that I learned that Corpus Christi is a three-hour drive from the hotel I'd booked. The weather was dreadful. Corpus Christi had snow for the first time in 110 years, and he only got to windsurf one day. But he did catch up on his sleep, and the time away really seemed to help. I cite this example because it also illustrates how important humor is for relieving stress.)

There may be times when your care partner just needs a break for a day or two, or she may need to be away from you for other reasons, such as a business trip or a hospital stay. Both you and your care partner need to have activities in life that do not revolve around PD. However, your care needs do not stop when your care partner needs a break. If you are unable to handle the activities of daily living on your own, due to PD or some other health problem, this is where **respite care** comes into play.

Using respite care does not make you a "bad" care partner!

Some care partners feel guilty using respite care, because they feel they are letting down their loved one with Parkinson's. On the contrary, if occasional respite care helps keep your care partner happy, healthy, and loving, it's good for everyone.

Care partners may also feel like using respite care means they are complaining or that using respite care is spending money on a luxury. Again, I urge you to think of this as an investment in your relationship. I try to look at it from the point of view that anyone I pay to take care of me, or of my children, or of my parents, will expect time off. Why shouldn't care partners, who receive no money for their hard work, receive that same benefit?

There are two types of respite care, which is essentially adult day care. There's in-home care, where someone comes to your home to look after you, and there are respite facilities where you go to the facility for care. Some facilities offer only daytime programs. Others are equipped for overnight stays.

If you require only minimal assistance, in-home care may be the most cost-effective and easiest to organize. Outside facilities offer activities and socializing that are often missing from in-home care. Otherwise, the deciding factors are cost, availability, and personal preference.

In-home care

A growing number of companies and small businesses provide differing levels of in-home care, so choosing one all comes down to your individual needs. Some, such as the franchise-operated Right-At-Home, offer staff who will come into your home to assist with light housekeeping, take you grocery shopping and run errands, and provide companionship. They do not provide nursing or medical care and do not lift patients. Clients generally pay an hourly fee, which may be calculated based on income. The cost varies by geographic location.

Other businesses have available LPNs (licensed practical nurses), CNAs (certified nursing aides), or HHAs (home health aides) to offer assistance administering or overseeing medications and assist with bathing and other self care issues. Fees may be hourly or daily. The cost of these services also varies widely by location and may be based on income.

FINDING HOME CARE

If someone is going to be coming into your home, you will want to feel safe having that person around. When hiring through an agency, ask whether a background check has been done, and if so, review the results.

Ask for references from previous home-care clients as well as the aide's other jobs. For instance, you might be a bit apprehensive about hiring someone who has worked for twenty years in a factory and is now applying to work for you. Such a person may have a stellar performance record on the assembly line, but that is not the job that he will be doing for you.

If at all possible, you, as the person receiving care, and your care partner, who has to feel comfortable leaving you in someone else's care, should both interview applicants. It is critical that both of you trust and get along with this person.

Ideally, you will find someone who has experience dealing with people with Parkinson's disease. This may be difficult, though, particularly if you are in a rural area or far from a major city, so don't rule out candidates who don't have PD experience. They can do just as good a job caring for you as long as they're well trained.

Respite care programs or facilities

There are many more choices for care if you only need it during the workday, Monday through Friday. Senior centers, hospitals, nursing homes, and facilities dedicated to caring for people with PD or Alzheimer's disease offer adult daycare programs. If you will need overnight or weekend care, your choices drop dramatically.

Day programs are often scheduled like child care: morning, afternoon, or full-day care. Usually, there is a series of activities throughout the day, such as bingo, singing, and games. Meals are offered and there may be exercise programs, too.

Unfortunately, there are not many respite care programs that cater specifically to people with PD and offer overnight and weekend care. If this is what you need, get recommendations from your doctor, or from people in your support group. Check the Community/Human Resources section in your local phone book.

Obviously, you want to have more selection criteria for care programs than whatever happens to be the first listing in the phone book. Here are some factors to consider:

CHECKLIST FOR EVALUATING RESPITE CARE FACILITIES

Here are some key questions to ask when choosing a respite care facility:

- ✔ Is it near your home?
- ✔ Is it open 24 hours/day, 7 days/week? If not, what are the days and hours of operation?

✔ What is the capacity of the facility?

✔ What is the maximum ratio of staff to clients?

✔ Does the facility serve only families dealing with PD? If not, how likely is it that you would be the only Parkie there at any given time?

✔ Is the staff specifically trained to handle the needs of people with PD? Is all the staff trained, or just some?

✔ Is there a doctor on-site at all times? If not, what is their protocol for obtaining medical care for clients?

✔ How long has the facility been in business?

✔ What is the cost? Is there a sliding scale fee or reduced-cost option for lower-income families?

✔ Do they allow drop-in or last-minute care options? What sort of advance reservation is required?

✔ Is there a waiting list? If so, how long?

✔ Are there any beds kept available for emergencies?

✔ What is the staff turnover rate? (This can be an indicator that the facility is not well managed. If turnover is very high and you're going to be there on a frequent basis, you might want to ask the senior staff how they deal with training and consistency of care.)

✔ Do you know anyone who has used the facility? Can the facility provide any references? (For privacy reasons, the center cannot give you names of clients without prior permission, but frequently when there are satisfied clients, they will volunteer to serve as references.)

✔ When you visit (and you should visit before using the facility), do the clients seem happy, safe, engaged, and well supervised?

✔ Is the site clean, well maintained, and well lit?

✔ Does the staff check in daily with care partners, or is communication only "as needed"?

✔ What sorts of activities are provided for clients? (If I am going to be away from my home so that my husband can get a break, I don't want to just sit in a TV room and watch *Wheel of Fortune*. I expect some activity.

There are more questions that could be asked, but this list should get you and your care partner thinking about what you might look for in a facility.

An excellent online resource

The Northwest Parkinson's Foundation (NWFP) has a free online curriculum that is designed to help staff working in long-term care facilities to respond better to the needs of the people with Parkinson's disease who are in their care. Go to www.parkinsonseducator.org/ and check it out.

Respite care can be an important resource for both you and your care partner. Using respite services is an investment in keeping you both sane and as healthy as possible.

IN A SENTENCE:

> *Care partners need a break sometimes, and professional respite care is available to enable your care partner to take some time off without having to worry.*

learning

Nutrition

JUST AS it affects every other area of your life, PD will affect how and what you eat. Depression and anxiety may increase your appetite or take it away completely. Feeling self-conscious about tremors may also change what you eat. Muscle rigidity can impact every stage of eating: stiff fingers and hands may make it difficult to cut food or bring your fork or spoon to your mouth; tight throat muscles can lead to choking and swallowing problems; and rigid abdominal muscles can cause the stomach to empty more slowly and cause constipation. Tremors obviously can make cutting food tough, and eating soup is a nightmare! If PD has diminished your sense of smell or taken it away entirely, you will find that food doesn't taste as good (much of our sense of taste is actually based on the scent of the food) and you may not have much of an appetite.

Medication can have a big impact on your appetite

Medications can either make you nauseous and take away your appetite or, as is the case with many antidepressants, stimulate your appetite and cause considerable weight gain if not controlled. Eating many small meals throughout the day may help with both sides of the appetite spectrum. If medication is fueling your appetite, ask yourself whether it is really food you want, or something else.

Dyskinesia and tremors burn calories

Dyskinesia and tremors can burn an amazing number of calories while making it difficult to get food to your mouth, so choosing foods is even more important if you experience those symptoms. Don't go for empty calories. Eat whole grains and plenty of fruits and vegetables. If you need help with your food choices, ask your doctor for a referral to a dietician or use the "Ask the Dietician" discussion forum on the National Parkinson Foundation Web site at www.parkinson.org/.

Using a straw can help liquids—including soups—reach their intended target. Travel mugs with lids can also serve as an adult "sippy cup" to avoid spills.

Protein may affect Levodopa effectiveness

For some, eating a food high in protein too close to your Sinemet dose—usually less than thirty minutes after your medication—can affect your body's absorption of the drug. When I first began taking Sinemet, I had no problems with protein. It has been in the last eighteen months or so that I have noticed that I really do need to avoid protein until my evening meal. In other words, I had more than five years where it made no difference. Protein consumption is another thing to track in your drug diary.

Some foods are choking hazards

Choosing foods that are the right consistency is very important for those who have choking problems. If you have had choking episodes, you may want to check into having a "swallow study" done. This test will help to determine which types of foods are more apt to make you choke and provide guidance on what forms your food should take. For some people, liquids make them choke, so energy or protein drinks would be a bad idea. For others, dry, crumbly foods will catch in their throats and bring on bouts of coughing or choking.

Some nutrients are particularly important

Some nutrients are even more important for people with Parkinson's than for the average healthy person. For instance, people with PD have a higher risk of bone-thinning, which can lead to fractures if you fall. To avoid developing osteoporosis, be sure to get plenty of calcium, magnesium, and vitamins K and D in your diet. Many dairy products and even such items as orange juice are available with added calcium and vitamin D. Sunlight is another source of vitamin D. Magnesium and calcium help to control the contraction and relaxation of our muscles.

British physician Geoffrey Leader recommends that people with PD have their mineral levels checked. His research indicates that we may be deficient in some minerals that are very important for our bodies to function properly. For example, many people with Parkinson's are deficient in zinc, and zinc is needed to metabolize protein. (This makes me wonder whether a zinc deficiency may play any role in the excess formation of alpha-synuclein, a protein that is believed to play a role in the development of PD.)

Manganese is another mineral many of us are lacking, and manganese is necessary to our metabolism of certain essential fatty acids. On the other hand, we do know that too much manganese is linked to parkinsonism, especially in welders.

Vitamins, minerals, and herbal supplements

Ideally, we would be able to get all of the nutrients that our bodies need from the foods that we eat. Realistically, though, we may need some help. Many health-care providers recommend that people with Parkinson's take a daily multivitamin.

Calcium supplements can also be helpful in keeping our bones strong, which is important since our risk of falling is greater than the average person.

Vitamins C and E are antioxidants, which destroy free radicals, a possible cause of damage to dopaminergic neurons. Don't go overboard, though. Too much vitamin C (more than 2,000 milligrams/day) can irritate your stomach and cause diarrhea. Vitamin E is stored in fat and thus can build up to toxic levels, so don't take more than 1,000 milligrams/day (this is the equivalent of 1,500 international units [IUs] from natural sources or 1,100 IUs from synthetic sources of vitamin E). Most nutritional supplements contain 400 IU per pill. Too much vitamin E can also interfere with blood-thinner medications.[1]

GET YOUR B'S

Vitamins B_6, B_{12}, and folic acid (folate), which are known collectively as B-complex vitaims, are all very important in your diet.[2] B_6 is necessary for hormone and neurotransmitter production as well as protein formation. When you need energy, vitamin B_6 releases your body's stored sugar.

Vitamin B_{12} is important for DNA synthesis and in creation of red blood cells and the protective membrane around nerve cells called the myelin sheath. Vitamin B_{12} is especially important for seniors, as it's been estimated that 42 percent of all seniors over age sixty-five may have a B_{12} deficiency.[3] If you are concerned that you may have a vitamin deficiency, see if your doctor will refer you to a dietician, or consult one of the publications listed in the Resources section.

Folic acid (folate) works with B_{12} in DNA synthesis. Together, the "three B's" help to clear the bloodstream of **homocysteine,** which is an amino acid. Overabundance of homocysteine has been implicated in causing heart attacks, stroke, and dementia. In PD the compound is suspected of damaging DNA in the substantia nigra, where dopamine is produced.

If you ingest too much B_6—more than 15 milligrams per day—it can interfere with Sinemet absorption, so you need to pay attention to your B_6 intake.

Don't forget to drink water!

While most of us don't think of water as "food," some of our daily water intake does come from food. Water is extremely critical to proper functioning of our digestive and respiratory systems. It lubricates our joints and flushes waste products out of bloodstreams. Being dehydrated can even affect your balance and your mental state! Dehydration leads to thousands of hospital visits each year (not all of them are by PD patients). Many of the PD medications can increase the risk of dehydration, so it's vital that you keep yourself hydrated.

Some medications may cause edema (water retention and swelling), which can raise your blood pressure and your weight. If you notice that you are retaining water, tell your doctor and modify your salt intake. Sodium can make you retain even more water. Conversely, potassium, which is found in bananas and other fruits and vegetables, helps your body to rid itself of excess water and toxins.

Where to go for help

If you have questions about how you might want to modify your diet to deal with your PD, ask your health-care provider to refer you to a dietician who has experience with Parkinson's patients. The national PD groups—the American Parkinson's Disease Association, the Parkinson's Disease Foundation, and the National Parkinson Foundation—all have free publications on PD and nutrition and have "Ask the Dietician" features on their Web sites.

IN A SENTENCE:

> *What and how much you eat can be affected by your medications, symptoms such as dyskinesias or tremors, and your mood.*

How PD May Affect the Power Balance of Family Life

PARKINSON'S DISEASE becomes an uninvited guest to all family dynamics and discussions. It will be your conjoined twin from now on, and although there will be times when its influence on your close relationships is benign, there will also be moments when PD squashes the wants and needs of your family members like a bug. In the past, you and your partner have probably worked out a system that allows the two of you to share responsibilities and decisions, from the mundane (housework, cooking, laundry) to the intimate (sex, child-rearing, finances). By recognizing the ways that PD can affect this balance of decision-making power and responsibility, you can hopefully head off some of the power struggles or burnout that could otherwise occur.

Managing your money—whose job is it?

Perhaps you have been the one in your household to keep track of the finances. Your spouse has had little or no role in paying bills, balancing the checkbook, tracking investments. You know that it is both fiscally prudent and practical to show your partner how to handle these tasks, but you find yourself feeling that if you do this, you will be losing control over a very important part of your life. You may feel like a child who has to ask for your allowance. You may also feel that your Parkinson's has affected your ability to contribute to the management of the household and that you do not deserve money to spend on your own needs or enjoyment. Conversely, your care partner may feel unprepared or unqualified to handle your financial situation. Or she may feel resentful that this is one more very large burden that she would prefer not to undertake.

I wish that I could offer more suggestions beyond having routine conversations about money and consulting a financial adviser. Alas, there is no "finance fairy" to come around once a month to take care of your bills. I can say from personal experience that lack of attention to this matter can be devastating.

Drowning in paperwork

As if managing money isn't enough of a challenge to begin with, finding ways to finance PD can complicate things even more. Parkinson's treatment is expensive, even for those who have earned a good income or saved a considerable sum for their retirement. Merely keeping track of the expenses and whether or not they are covered by insurance or Medicare is quite a task. Making appointments, managing their paperwork, and submitting receipts can seem like a full-time job. When you have Parkinson's, you may find it difficult to concentrate or focus on these chores, but you don't want to admit to your care partner that this is happening. Giving up control can be very difficult. Meanwhile, the care partner is most likely thinking, "I really don't have time for this." But someone needs to do it, or you will have a real mess on your hands.

Paul and I try to share the responsibility. I do what I can to keep track of receipts and bills and sort them. He deals with paying bills, which we do electronically. If paperwork, such as Explanation of Benefits forms from our health insurance company, requires phone calls for more information or follow-up (they want to pay as little as possible to the least number of providers, so they do not make resolving questions easy), I do that, because

I am home during the day. This system will not work for everyone, but hopefully it will help you to think of possible scenarios that will work for you.

Safety concerns

For us Parkies, it is a blow to the ego to admit that we are worried about our ability to drive safely or use sharp knives or climb ladders to complete home repairs. It is an even bigger blow to be told by someone else that you can't do these things. Whenever possible, you need to stop and think about how long it might take you to recover if you get into a car accident or fall from a ladder, and let someone else do these things. As Paul put it: "If you think mobility is bad now, try it on crutches!" For care partners, it is helpful if you work with the person with Parkinson's to make sure there are things that he can do to feel like a productive member of the household.

Housing

Speaking of households, you may have thought that your current living space would be where you would live out your twilight years—and it still might be. But now is a good time to start discussing the what-ifs about housing. It is much better to discuss possible future scenarios now, when you are in control of the circumstances, than when your needs become urgent. For instance, if you wait five years to have your home evaluated for accessibility and safety and suddenly you need to add a ramp, you may find that your apartment building can't or won't accommodate you in a timely manner.

When you are discussing housing, you should talk about your geographic location as well. If you have just been diagnosed with PD at age sixty-two and you had planned to retire to Florida when you hit sixty-five, maybe you should do it now. Or perhaps you'll want to move closer to your children so that you can spend as much time with them as possible now, while you're healthier. And they'll be closer by when you need them.

"Do I look like a chauffeur to you?"

PD can take away your autonomy in another way: by preventing you from driving. For many of us, this will occur at some point. It may be because of PD; it could be failing eyesight due to aging. However it happens, losing your seat behind the wheel is a great blow to your independence and to your care partner's as well. Think about this: there are still many women of a certain age who never learned to drive; they relied on their husbands to drive them.

Losing your ability to drive is like being demoted to junior high and having to either whine your way into getting a ride to the mall from your mom, or charm your way into a seat with your big brother to go to the movies. It can be very demoralizing to have to ask for a service that you have provided for yourself for so long.

For care partners, it means extra stress, too—they in essence become our chauffeurs, driving us everywhere we have to go and running extra errands because we can't do them.

For those who have always relied on public transit, your mode of transportation may have to change. For instance, you may find that you're unable to walk all the way to the bus stop or climb the steps to the subway station anymore.

Help around the house

Who does what around the house is already contentious enough in many American households today, without adding a chronic illness to the mix. Each family has its own way of dealing with housework, so I won't try to impose one on you. Just be aware that at some point, your PD is bound to have an impact on the division of labor in the housekeeping department. You may find it easier to hire a cleaning person for general basic housecleaning or specific/seasonal tasks if no one on the care team really relishes performing such duties.

Don't sweat the small stuff

Housework, bookkeeping, driving—all these things are part of your everyday life, and when you begin to have problems in these areas, it is very likely due to larger issues that you are not facing as a couple or as a family. And if you don't discuss it now and again, resentment around these topics can build and fester.

Here are some of the bigger issues that cause problems for all Parkies at one time or another:

Guilt. Feelings of guilt can weigh on a relationship like bags of cement. When you have a chronic illness like Parkinson's disease, it is common to feel guilty because "I let the family down," "All of our hopes and dreams will never come true," "I can't be a good wife and mother," and so on. All sorts of self-deprecating messages play over and over in our head.

Meanwhile, your care partner may be feeling guilty because "I'm healthy and he's not, so I shouldn't go out and have fun with my friends," "I want to be able to do all those things we planned to do together, and I don't know if she still wants to do them." You get the picture.

Resentment. Feeling guilty is no fun, so you may move on to resentment, which is much more fun for your ego. Your feelings of resentment may not even be directed toward your partner; you may just be mad at the world for being stuck in this predicament.

Anxiety. People with PD are prone to anxiety anyway, but now you may be worrying about whether your partner will still find you attractive as your PD worsens, will she still love you, will he be able to care for you, and so on. All of these are very common issues that concern most of us with Parkinson's.

Care partners may very well be asking themselves the same questions. And the only way that either side is going to get answers is to talk. It may not be a fun conversation, and it may not be short. It might not end happily, but if you don't try, all you will have is that icky, hot, but clammy, nauseating, unsettled feeling of uncertainty.

We can easily let our feelings build until somebody explodes

If you allow your feelings of guilt to keep you from telling your partner how guilty you feel, the whole cycle goes on and on until something brings it to a head. Usually it is something that under any other circumstances would hardly be worth mentioning. Instead, you end up thinking ,"I cannot spend another minute of my life with this person!" because you have let the pressure of your feelings build up to their flash point. If you don't manage the situation, your relationship can be devastated.

Create your own "warning system" for your relationship with your care partner. Don't let anger, guilt, and resentment build up to the point that they could wash away your feelings of love for each other.

A Care Partner's Perspective

I ASKED Angela, a care partner whose husband was diagnosed at age twenty-three, to think about how she and Karl have maintained a healthy relationship. She made some good suggestions about how to deal with Parkinson's and marriage, and about how care partners can maintain their own identity:

○ Love the person, not the disease. You can love the person and absolutely hate PD. PD is not part of the person's character, personality, or ability to love.

○ Live life for the moment and make the most out of each day.

○ Get involved with a care partner support group where you can share experiences and build a support network. There's a lot to be learned from those who have walked before you.

○ Be patient and flexible! PD makes every day a different day; no two days are the same.

○ Make sure to take time for yourself. Even if you not performing daily care giving (activities of daily living) of your loved one with PD, make sure you have time for yourself. Get out to lunch with friends. Get involved with social groups (non-PD). Take time for your favorite hobby. This helps you to keep your sanity.

IN A SENTENCE:

> *You and your care partner must work together to deal with the changes that PD brings to your relationship.*

learning

PD Isn't Just for Older People Anymore

FOR ME, the path from the first sign of Parkinson's disease to actually receiving a diagnosis took nearly eighteen months. My situation is far from unique. In fact, my diagnosis was downright speedy compared to that of Pam, who was diagnosed at thirty-seven—fifteen years after she first noticed symptoms!

Differences between young-onset and typical PD

There are a few differences in the way that Parkinson's disease affects younger people (those diagnosed before age fifty-five) and older "typical" patients (those fifty-five or older at diagnosis).

"PRESENTING" SYMPTOMS
Younger patients are more likely to show signs of bradykinesia (slowness of movement) as an initial symptom of PD, while older patients are more likely to experience tremor. Those with young-onset Parkinson's disease may also report a burning/

stinging/tingling sensation (paraesthesia) in their hands and feet. This symptom is rare in older people with Parkinson's.

A longitudinal study done in Australia found that older people were diagnosed sooner after noticing symptoms, but their disease tended to progress more quickly after the disease was discovered.[1] I can think of a few reasons why older patients might be diagnosed more quickly: so many physicians still think that PD is an "old person's disease," and as we age, we expect things in our body to start to deteriorate and notice them earlier.

Medication issues

Treating young-onset PD poses special challenges to pharmaceutical companies and medical device manufacturers. For instance, people with YOPD (we often refer to ourselves in written materials as "YOPDers") may still be having children and nursing babies. Therefore, it is imperative that drug manufacturers, regulatory agencies, and health-care providers be sure that PD medications are safe for women of childbearing age, are not excreted in breast milk, and are not linked to birth defects or other health problems in children of mothers (or fathers) who have taken the medication. If there is little or no information about the potential health risks, your physician needs to have a frank discussion with you so that you can weigh the benefits of the medication with the risks to your child.

UNKNOWN SIDE EFFECTS

People with YOPD are likely to be on medications for much longer than folks who are diagnosed in their sixties or seventies. We need to know the health risks of being on Sinemet for ten, fifteen, or twenty years. What happens to the brain after ten or more years of deep-brain stimulation? These are questions that are largely unanswered, because the majority of treatments have been created for, or marketed to, geriatric patients.

RESISTANCE TO TAKING MEDICATIONS

Maybe it is because we are in denial, still wanting to feel young and "bullet-proof," but a lot of YOPDers are very resistant to taking meds. Sometimes we wait until a fall or some other event slaps us upside the head to get our attention. Almost invariably, once we finally surrender and begin a drug regimen, we wish we had started it sooner. Roberta, diagnosed at age forty-four, recalls,

> I didn't want to take any medications. I said that I was okay; I could wait. After starting Amantadine, I could not believe the difference in my life. Why did I fight taking it so long? I was allowing myself to curl up and sleep from all the fatigue. Now I look at PD as a hurdle in my life, some physical difficulties that I have to learn to overcome. I am enjoying my life more than ever before. My life and my family have greater meaning to me.

Dyskinesia is nearly inevitable

For some reason, young Parkies appear doomed to get dyskinesia. As I mentioned on page 40, the rate of dyskinesia within the first three years on Sinemet is 74 percent in YOPDers.

Lack of financial preparation

Those of us who are diagnosed before fifty-five are much more likely to still be working—we may not even have reached our peak earning potential. With fewer years worked, our individual retirement accounts (IRAs) are smaller and our Social Security benefit checks will be smaller. We are more likely to still be making mortgage payments and to have children in school or college.

Years of medication costs—and potentially, surgical expenses, too—can add significant debt load. We may not have saved quite as much as we would have liked for travel and other benefits of retirement.

More likely to be raising children

People with young-onset PD may not have even begun their families, let alone finished raising their children. There is very little information available on the potential effects of Parkinson's medications on fertility, pregnancy, and nursing, nor are there many studies on the implications for birth defects. These are extremely difficult personal choices that young couples affected by PD may wish to discuss with a therapist, as well as their physician.

Keeping up with young children or grandchildren is a challenge for able-bodied adults. For parents with PD, that challenge is magnified by mobility issues, work, and other factors.

On the brighter side

People with YOPD are likely to be healthier and have good mobility when diagnosed. You have to deal with PD, but that may be your only disease. Seniors could be contending with several ailments at one time.

Younger people with Parkinson's have a much lower risk of developing dementia. Depression and mental health issues have had less stigma attached to them in recent generations, so young Parkies often feel more comfortable seeking treatment for such problems.

Realistically, people with early-onset PD have a better chance of living to see and benefit from a cure. I am not suggesting that older patients should abandon hope. However, I do think that it's important that we all understand that even if a cure for PD were found today, it would not be available tomorrow. In all likelihood, it would be a few years before it was widely available. So that is why I recommend emotionally living each day as if it were your last, but taking care of your body as if you were going to be using it forever.

IN A SENTENCE:

> *Many life circumstances, including work, children, and long-term financial stability, are different for people with young-onset PD.*

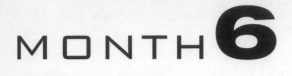

MONTH 6

living

When Adult Children Care for a Parent with PD

BEING THE spouse of someone with PD is difficult, but if you have grown children who may be involved in your care, they face their own unique set of challenges.

> I think just learning about the disease helped me cope with my father's diagnosis. I didn't know a thing about PD at the time and wasn't sure how PD would affect him. I was very scared, and reading more helped me understand what the future held. —KIM, *care partner, whose father has had PD for more than eight years*

Many people with PD come to rely on their adult children for care, whether it is because their spouse or partner has passed away or is incapacitated, or because their son or daughter is best equipped to provide help.

In many societies, it is simply understood that children take care of their parents when they reach old age. It is done out of gratitude for the sacrifices that parents have made to provide food, shelter, clothing, and education for their children and out of recognition of the wisdom and tradition that elders can continue to share with their families. Indeed, most of the immigrants who arrive in this country come here with a history of living with their extended families. Several generations of Americans have not been raised in that tradition, however, and so may view taking in a parent as an imposition rather than an honor. Due to factors such as Social Security benefits, relative affluence in the latter half of the twentieth century, and the globalization of the economy, seniors have been less likely to live in the same city as their children. Comparatively few have lived in the same house as their grown children and grandchildren.

Now, with the soaring costs of health-care, prescription drugs, and housing, older Americans with PD are in a tough spot. You have gotten used to your independence. You like having your own home. You like peace and quiet. You like watching the grandchildren when it is your choice. And your children like their space, their things, and their privacy as well.

This cultural change can make it awkward for seniors with PD to ask their kids for help, whether they need a ride to a doctor's appointment, a place to live, or money for medication.

Physical distance and busy schedules, two-parent households where both work, and one-parent households where a single person juggles parenting and career—all of these things compete for attention in the minds of grown children who have parents living with Parkinson's, who may not stop to think very often about Mom or Dad.

Discussing your disease with your adult children

Talking about PD with your adult children is a mixed blessing. On the one hand, they will have a much better chance of understanding the answers you give to their questions. On the other hand, adult children can sometimes feel too embarrassed to ask the questions that are really on their minds.

If at all possible, tell your kids about your disease in person. That way they can see how you are doing, and you can get a better sense of their reactions.

Have a "family meeting" to discuss what your doctor has told you so far regarding your disease, how you are feeling physically and emotionally, what your treatment plans are, and how your various family members feel. This does not mean that you should allow your children to tell you how to handle the treatment of your disease.

Respect their feelings

When I talk with my family about my PD and my son says he feels afraid when he watches me lift pots off the stove, his feeling is valid. So are my feelings of disappointment and sadness that he has these concerns. Does that mean that I need to give up cooking on the stove? Not necessarily. I need to separate his feelings and reasoning from mine. In this case, we have reached a compromise: I have agreed to ask my husband to lift heavy pots from the stove for me, if he is available. I also received a pair of silicone oven mitts to make lifting hot pots safer for anyone.

Do your best to respect how your children feel about PD and how it's affecting you, even if you don't agree with them. Mutual respect will be a key factor in maintaining strong relationships as you live through your illness.

It's okay to not have all the answers to their questions

You do not have to be able to answer all of their questions. After all, Parkinson's is a complicated illness and even your doctor may not have all the answers to your questions. Since the disease is going to affect you all in one way or another, you can agree to learn about it together.

Your children can be valuable resources

It is normal to feel, "I am the parent; I am supposed to know how to handle this." In this ever-changing world, we are all learning how to handle new situations all of the time. Your children may be able to help you to learn how to use a computer in order to get current PD information or to participate in an online support group. Doing things the "modern" way does not necessarily make them better or the right options for you, but your children can be a big help if you choose to go down that road.

Strive for a care partner relationship with your children

You may be worried that by depending on your children for things, whether it is information, housing, or transportation, you will have to defer to their wishes about your treatment. You are all adults now, but it can be difficult to treat each other as peers or equals. We have grown so accustomed to the unequal balance of power in a parent-child relationship that in situations where grown children have more skills or information, they can wind up treating us like children. We may also feel childlike or immature because of our lack of knowledge.

Operate from the standpoint that you are still very much in control of your faculties and that you can make your own decisions, and demand that respect from your children. It is true that some of us will go on to develop dementia and will forfeit at least a portion of our decision-making power, but a PD diagnosis doesn't mean you sign over your autonomy to anyone.

A note to grown children who care for parents with PD

Your mother or father has been diagnosed with a brain disease. Of course you are concerned and want to help. Please keep in mind that this diagnosis does not automatically mean your parent will develop dementia or that he or she will have to come and live with you. (He or she may not want to live with you.)

The first thing to do is to learn more about how your parent is doing now. If you are reading this book, you will have some sense of what to look for in terms of symptoms and behaviors. Some parents are more forthcoming with information than others. Your mom or dad may be too proud or too concerned about burdening you to tell you how they are really doing or to ask for help. In that case, you may have to go on a "fishing expedition." Call and ask Dad how he is doing. Invite Mom over for dinner or for a visit (but don't expect her to cook or watch the grandkids). Let your parent know that you have been doing some reading on PD and want to see how his or her disease compares with what you've read. You might also ask Dad if you can accompany him to his next doctor's appointment. If he is resistant, show him the section in this book that talks about how helpful it can be to have someone along who will take notes at appointments.

Once you get more information about your parent's prognosis—either from him or her directly or from the doctor—you need to think about how you would like to be involved and the level of commitment that you can realistically make.

When you have some sense of what you could do, have a talk with Mom or Dad. If I were facing this situation with my dad, I would say something like, "You know, Dad, I'm really worried about you. It seems like you are falling a lot, and even though I don't see any bones poking out of your skin, I am worried that you are hurting yourself. I think it would be a good idea to tell your neurologist about this. You are a grownup and can make your own decisions, but I hope that you will see your doctor. I want my sons to have their grandpa around for many years to come. I love you and I will do whatever I can to help. I need you to tell me what that might be." There—I've said my piece and been honest and straightforward. I don't think I have been disrespectful. In fact, in order to be respectful, I must accept his decision. This may not be easy if he declines my offer, but I will have done what I would like him to do for me.

The golden rule applies to families, too

What I'm saying to all care partners is treat the person with PD just as you would your very best friend in the whole world. And we Parkies should regard our care partners the same way. Of course there's comfort in knowing that you "should" always have a place with your family, but wouldn't we all rather be welcomed like a cherished friend? It all comes down to treating others the way we would like to be treated.

IN A SENTENCE:

> *When you require care from your adult children to help you cope with your PD, your family dynamics will change.*

learning

Talking to Young Kids about PD

MANY OF us with PD are frequently around children. They could be our own kids, grandchildren, kids we teach, or children from our neighborhood. We don't often give them credit, but they nearly always know it if something is amiss with our health or if there is "something going on" in the family.

Answer their questions

Children—especially young children—are blessed with an innocent honesty that allows them to ask the questions that are usually on everyone's mind. By answering their questions as best you can, you can let the kids know that there is nothing shameful about having PD. (It can be embarrassing, yes, but not shameful.) They will be more likely to want to be near you and to help as your disease progresses. If your child or grandchild is taught to think that Parkinson's is something that we whisper about and try to hide, he or she could think that PD is "bad," contagious, or their fault. I know that I do not want my sons feeling that way about my disease.

When we educate children about Parkinson's disease, we are teaching the next generations of doctors, nurses, social workers, attorneys, researchers—members of our society that could help to find a cure or care for us in later stages of the disease. If we have taught them that PD is something they shouldn't talk about or that it is not important, we have lost an opportunity to raise compassionate, caring people. They may decide that we do not deserve certain medical benefits or social programs, that research for a cure is not necessary.

Tough questions from real kids

My older son was six when I was diagnosed with PD, so he has very few memories of me as a "normal" mom. My son Bennett has never known me without PD. My husband and I have always encouraged them to ask any questions they have and to let us know what they think about how the disease is affecting our family.

I have talked about my PD in each of my sons' classrooms. Bennett is in second grade, and at that age children don't filter their questions; they just ask or say whatever is on their minds. Here is a list of questions (and my answers) that arose during a presentation I made about my PD volunteer work to a group of about thirty first- and second-graders. Hopefully, this will help you answer some questions the kids in your life may ask you.

Do you have trouble getting dressed?
Yes, I do sometimes. That is why I generally don't wear clothes with a lot of buttons; I wear shirts or dresses that I can just pull over my head. Zippers can be difficult, too. Pull-on pants are very helpful. Sometimes I need help getting dressed.

Do they know what causes it?
No one knows what causes Parkinson's disease. I believe my disease was caused by being exposed to a lot of pesticides—chemicals used to kill bugs or weeds—when I was younger. But no one knows for sure.

Do they know how to cure it?
No, right now no one knows how to cure Parkinson's disease. I take a lot of medicine throughout the day to help me from getting too stiff. Some of that medicine is what makes me so wiggly.

Do you get into a lot of car accidents?
[I was very dyskinetic, fidgeting in my seat, which I'm sure is why this question was asked.] No, but I could if I were to try to drive very far when I'm wiggly like this. If I am like this, I get someone else to drive, and there will be a time soon when it's not safe for me or for other people if I drive.

Do you shake sometimes?
Yes, sometimes, but my main symptom is being stiff. Some people shake a lot. Parkinson's disease affects each person a little differently.

Do you have trouble tying your shoes?
Yes, I do sometimes, so I wear shoes that don't need to be tied, or I ask for help.

I also spoke to my son Alex's class of seventh- and eighth-graders. When I asked Alex's permission to speak to his class, he had warned me that his classmates might find it too awkward or embarrassing to ask questions while I was there, so his teacher and I agreed that leaving out a question box after my visit might be the best approach. However, I was pleasantly surprised at the kids' willingness to posit questions during my hour in the classroom. Here are some of their questions:

Are your children more likely to get Parkinson's because you have it?
Yes, my kids have a slightly higher risk of developing PD.

Do you "wiggle" while you sleep?
Before last year, I would have said no. However, I had a sleep study done last year because I had been snoring and my husband thought I might have sleep apnea like he does. I do not have sleep apnea, but the technician who did my study said that I was moving my legs quite a bit. I do not seem to feel more tired as a result.

Is it hard to type or write?
Yes. My handwriting has never been all that legible, but there are times now when even I can't read it. It has gotten somewhat smaller, but I have not exhibited the very tiny, cramped handwriting known as micrographia. When I am very stiff, or if my dyskinesia is bad, writing or typing are nearly impossible.

Tell them what they need to know

Use age-appropriate language. If you are responding to a three-year-old's question about why Grandpa's hand is shaking, telling her about the lack of adequate dopamine in Grandpa's substantia nigra will not get the point across.

Young children have many misconceptions about the causes and duration of diseases like PD.

One of the first things you should explain to kids is that Parkinson's disease is NOT contagious! They cannot contract or spread the disease by being around you. However, because kids are used to personally dealing with contagious illnesses of short duration, don't be surprised if your child says at some point in the future, "You STILL have Parkinson's? Why isn't it gone?"

Second, it is critical that they know that nothing they have done caused your PD, and although they will want to do something to make it go away, loving you and spending time with you are the best medicines until a cure is found.

Dispense information in small doses

Kids have a way of letting you know that they have absorbed as much as they can on a topic for the time being. It is called "changing the subject." If your six-year-old granddaughter says, "Nana, why do your hands shake?" and you explain that you have a sickness that makes your brain send the wrong information to your muscles, that you take medicine to make you shake less, and that this is not a sickness that she can catch from you, she may say, "Okay. Can I have some ice cream?" When that happens, just let it go. Your granddaughter will surely ask more questions in the future when she's ready to hear more, and she'll probably even ask the same questions more than once.

A new resource for kids' PD information

Rasheda Ali, daughter of world champion boxer Muhammad Ali, has just published a wonderful book for kids called *I'll Hold Your Hand So You Won't Fall: A Child's Guide to Parkinson's Disease*. This is a book for adults to read to their children or grandchildren. It uses multicultural photos and illustrations and questions or statements from kids on specific aspects of Parkinson's disease, such as tremors, slurred speech, depression, early stages of PD, and surgery. Each section also includes suggested questions for beginning a discussion with a child about the topic, a fact or two, and definitions of PD-related words and phrases (e.g., tremor, dyskinesia, stooped posture, exercise.

This book will help to fill gaps in information for children and also for people of color.

A *very special prescription*

When my older son, Alex, was about ten, I brought him with me to an appointment with my neurologist. (I can't remember why; he must have been out of school for some reason.) He watched and listened very patiently as I did all of my "party tricks" for Dr. Tuite. At the end of the appointment, the doctor asked Alex if he had any questions. He asked, "When are they going to find a cure?" Dr. Tuite did something that I will never forget. He explained that there were doctors and scientists working very hard to find a cure for Parkinson's, but until one is found, the best that Alex could do would be to give his mom a hug every day and tell her that he loves her. Here is a copy of that prescription:

Humor—potent medicine

Sometimes laughing and making fun of myself is the only alternative to having a complete meltdown, and if I have to do one or the other in public, I will take the laughter any time. I can always cry later in private.

Dyskinesia often provides an opportunity to laugh. Even now I'm sure that I am dyskinetic far more than I realize. Stress and nervousness makes it much worse, so whenever I am doing any public speaking, I always begin my remarks by explaining that I have Parkinson's disease and that the "dancing" the audience members will see me doing is a result of the medication and stage fright. I encourage them to move along with me if it will make them feel better, or to close their eyes and listen if my movements are too visually distracting.

If you are able to laugh at yourself and at the disease, your children will learn that you can have Parkinson's disease and still enjoy life. They will feel much more comfortable coming to you with questions, and you can all deal with them together. If the kids sense that PD is something to be ashamed of, they will probably assume that they should be ashamed, too, and that talking about PD is not okay.

So talk to your kids. Make sure they understand (as much as they can) what Parkinson's disease is and how it affects you. It's the best way to help your kids cope with your condition and maintain a strong family relationship.

IN A SENTENCE:

> Kids are very aware of your physical and emotional state, so it is important to discuss your PD with them in ways that are appropriate for their age and stage of emotional development.

HALF-YEAR MILESTONE

*Six months have gone by already, and you're probably begin-
ning to grow accustomed to the unpredictable nature of
Parkinson's disease.*

○ YOU HAVE LEARNED HOW PD CAN AFFECT
YOUR EATING HABITS, AND THE IMPORTANCE
OF INCLUDING MANY VITAMINS AND MINER-
ALS IN YOUR DIET.

○ YOU KNOW THAT PD CAN PROFOUNDLY
CHANGE YOUR RELATIONSHIPS WITH FAM-
ILY AND FRIENDS, AND YOU NOW HAVE
SOME TOOLS FOR ADDRESSING THOSE
CHALLENGES.

○ YOU CAN TALK TO YOUR CHILDREN AND
GRANDCHILDREN ABOUT PARKINSON'S DIS-
EASE AND ENCOURAGE THEM TO KEEP ASK-
ING QUESTIONS THAT YOU CAN ANSWER
TOGETHER.

Exercise

RESEARCH HAS shown that regular exercise (three to five times per week) and stretching can slow the advancement of PD symptoms. It can also help reduce stiffness, give you more energy, help your posture, and even be a social activity. Regular exercise can increase the levels of endorphins (the natural anti-depressant chemicals that your brain makes) and help you feel better about yourself.

Nearly everyone who completed my survey emphasized the importance of exercise and stretching—the sooner you begin, the better. Even if you do not consider yourself an athletic person and were not active before PD, it is not too late to start.

Check with your doctor

ALWAYS check with your health-care provider before beginning an exercise regime. She can let you know if there are types of activities to avoid or ones that would be especially beneficial.

Don't push yourself too hard

If you haven't been exercising, don't go out this afternoon and attempt to walk five miles, play several sets of tennis, or go rollerblading. If you ran a nine-minute mile in your thirties and are now in your sixties, don't expect you'll be able to do it now on the first day of your exercise program.

If the activity you are doing causes pain, stop! The 1980s Nike motto, "No pain, no gain," does not apply to people with Parkinson's disease. You need to be extra careful not to overstress your body or put yourself in situations where you could hurt yourself or fall. And if your PD symptoms are active, don't exercise. Exercising when you're "off" can be painful and dangerous.

Stretch

Doing some simple stretching exercises before you begin any exercise routine is a good idea, even if all you are going to do is walk around the block. Do your stretches slowly and gently; don't bounce. Your muscles are already tight, and pushing them too far without any preparation will only lead to pain, which means that you won't exercise, and then you'll have to contend with the pain from greater muscle rigidity.

Your doctor or a physical therapist can recommend stretching exercises and show you how to do them properly. Be sure to perform a variety of stretches that involve your entire body. This will help you to avoid developing problem areas.

Start your day every day by stretching. There are a number of stretching exercises that have been modified to be done from sitting or prone (lying flat) positions, so you can even do them before you get out of bed in the morning!

It is also a good idea to stretch again after you have completed your exercise routine.

Give yourself plenty of room

PD affects our spatial skills—that is, our ability to perceive the distance between objects. For instance, I have trouble gauging the distance between my body and a doorway or a wall. So if you're exercising in your living room, make sure you've cleared enough space around you to perform all the moves properly.

Aerobic exercise is important

The American College of Sports Medicine defines aerobic exercise as "any activity that uses large muscle groups, can be maintained continuously, and is rhythmic in nature."[1] By "continuously," they mean for a period of about twenty minutes. The point is to increase your heart rate and your breathing in order to strengthen your heart, build up your endurance, and make you stronger and more flexible.

There are two kinds of aerobic exercise: low-impact (easier on your bones and joints, because you have one foot on the ground at all times) and high-impact (includes jumping motions or other movements that can jar your body). Walking at your regular pace or climbing stairs are examples of low-impact exercises. Jogging or walking briskly, rowing, cross-country skiing, and using exercise equipment (treadmill, stationary bike, elliptical) are all high-impact activities. Talk to your doctor about which type of exercise is best for you.

Are you a team player, or do you do better "flying solo"?

Some of us had traumatic T-ball experiences as children and have avoided any and all group or team athletic activities since that time. Any number of exercise activities can be done alone, on your own time, in a place of your own choosing. Or perhaps you feel most energetic when you are in a group. Again, you have plenty of options, such as ballroom dancing, softball, golf, badminton, and hiking. Many exercise activities can be done both individually and as a group.

Here are some tips to help you get started on your exercise regimen:

Start slowly. Remember, Parkinson's disease affects our unconscious/automatic movements as well as our speed. You may find yourself having to think about where each foot will go next or counting dance steps. So start out nice and easy, doing fifteen to twenty minutes of activity, two or three days a week. Then, as you get stronger and more used to working out, increase the frequency and duration of your exercise.

Make it a routine. Walking twenty minutes one day and then jogging for ten minutes two weeks later will not provide a benefit. You need to be consistent with the amount of exercise you're getting each week.

Exercise to music. I have found that listening to upbeat music while I exercise is extremely helpful. I move at a consistent pace and it provides a pleasant distraction. I can even do voice exercises at the same time by singing along!

Do not exercise immediately after eating. There is a nugget of truth to the warning that we received as children: "Don't go swimming for at least an hour after you have eaten, or you will get stomach cramps and drown!" Working out after a heavy meal may cause nausea or vomiting. Most people generally do not feel their most energetic after a meal anyway, so plan your workouts accordingly.

Do not exercise right before bedtime. Exercise stimulates the muscles and gets your adrenaline going, which is not ideal at bedtime, when you want to be able to relax.

Do something you enjoy. Choose and activity that you really like—or at least you don't despise—doing. If your physician recommends walking thirty minutes each day, but to you that is as dull as watching paint dry, suggest another activity. Dancing, perhaps? Aerobics? Yoga? Racquetball?

Don't go it alone. Don't swim, hike, climb, sail, or engage in aerobic exercise completely alone or away from others. Like it or not, PD—even early PD—puts you at a higher risk for falls and fall-related injuries. It may be difficult to swallow your pride, but your life could depend upon it.

If the solo exercise you enjoy takes you away from areas where you can be seen or heard by others should you need medical attention, and you cannot or will not change your plans, be sure to let someone know where and when you are going and when to expect you back. Always carry a cell phone for emergencies.

Choosing an activity

If there is an activity that you engaged in prior to your diagnosis, chances are good that you can continue that pastime. You may need to modify your expectations of payoff at some point, but I know many people who have PD who regularly:

○ play racquetball or squash
○ play golf

- O   run
- O   walk
- O   hike
- O   bicycle
- O   rollerblade
- O   swim
- O   go ice-skating
- O   go dancing (ballroom, swing, line)

Swimming in particular is excellent exercise. It can be done at any age and does not require equipment per se. (Obviously, you need access to a pool or body of water.) If possible, swim in a heated pool; cold water can make your muscles contract and exacerbate rigidity.

If you are not self-directed—finding an exercise program

Many people are more apt to exercise if someone is there to instruct them on what to do. Your local YMCA/YWCA, community center, or neurology clinic may have classes designed especially for people with Parkinson's disease. Many community centers, hospitals, clinics, schools, or community colleges have general exercise classes or facilities available, and many of them have programs specifically for seniors as well.

If you are enrolling in a class that does not specifically target people with Parkinson's disease, be sure to inform the instructor of your condition and talk with him before the class starts to make sure he understands how Parkinson's affects the body. Also make sure that he understands that you may not be able to perform all of the exercises or activities that others in the class are able to do.

Care Partners Can Exercise, Too

Care partners are often encouraged to work out, too—not only to have a good understanding of how exercise can benefit their partner but also because it is critical for care partners to get exercise as well.

Home exercise equipment

Although they have taken a rap for sitting unused after purchase, home exercise machines can be a good way to ensure that you stick to your exercise routine. I have an elliptical machine in my family room. It has been a real godsend, allowing me to do my exercises at times that are convenient for me. I don't have to worry about whether the gym is open. I don't have to brush my teeth or comb my hair. I can wear whatever is comfortable for me, play the music of my choice, or watch TV or a movie.

Do not purchase any equipment unless you have discussed it with your doctor. Be sure that the equipment you choose allows you to do exercises that are appropriate for you, and that you are vigilant about keeping it in good working shape. The product should come with instructions on proper use and maintenance.

If you purchase used equipment (which can save you a considerable amount of money), do so from a retail store rather than at a rummage sale or from an individual. These stores sell products that are guaranteed to be in working order. They can also serve as a resource for how to operate the item.

IN A SENTENCE:

> *Exercise is a very important part of retaining your flexibility and strength, as well as reducing stress to keep your disease under control.*

learning

Traveling with PD

FOR MOST people with PD, particularly in the early stages of the disease, we can do all, or almost all, the things we did before. They may need to be modified for safety, or you may need to do them more slowly, but travel and other active hobbies can be continued—or started!—after you were told that you have PD.

On the road again—PD and driving

Rigidity, dyskinesia, and start hesitancy can affect your driving. You may back into things because you have difficulty turning to look over your shoulder, for example. You may rear-end other drivers at stop signs or intersections where traffic has slowed, because your reaction times aren't quick enough.

Because some symptoms of Parkinson's disease can be similar to those of intoxication or illegal drug use, it's a good idea to carry a card like the one below or information from your doctor explaining that you have Parkinson's disease.

MEDICAL ALERT

I have a condition called
PARKINSON'S DISEASE,
which makes me slow, and
sometimes I cannot
stand up or speak.

I AM NOT INTOXICATED
Please call my family or physician for help.

This wallet card is available from the National Parkinson Foundation and other organizations promoting PD awareness.

Getting a handicapped tag or plate

If you feel that Parkinson's disease may be affecting your driving or if it has affected your mobility, speak with your doctor about getting a handicapped tag or license plate for your car. Don't let pride get in your way. The tag or plate can be a blessing, especially if you live in a climate with weather extremes (high or low temperatures, snow, or rain). And remember that you are not required to park in a handicapped space. If you are feeling great and are confident that you will be able to make the trek back to the car after a couple of hours shopping at the mall, go for it!

Have your driving evaluated

You may not have noticed any changes yet, but your Parkinson's disease may already be affecting your ability to drive safely. Ask your care partner or other friends and loved ones to give you their honest evaluation. Have they noticed any changes or problems? Are they afraid to ride with you?

Many states have organizations that will assess your driving skills and let you know whether you should modify your driving habits or stop driving altogether. Consider this carefully and try to schedule an evaluation at a time when you are usually at your best. It is entirely possible that the evaluator may recommend that your license be revoked. If this happens, and you feel it has been done unfairly, speak with your doctor. Be candid with her about your driving habits and any symptoms that really would make you a danger on the road. I have some Parkie pals whose driving privileges had been revoked by driving evaluators but were reinstated with restrictions after intervention by their doctor.

Kimerly's story

KIMERLY, WHO was diagnosed at age thirty-three, tells of an incident in which she was driving to school to pick up her young son, who was six or seven years old at the time. She was experiencing some "off" time (her medication was not working optimally) and she was stopped by a highway patrolman who suspected her of driving while intoxicated.

Kim explained that she had Parkinson's disease and that this was why she was unable to pass the sobriety test (e.g., walking heel-to-toe in a straight line, saying the alphabet backward, and counting backward). He began writing her a ticket for driving under the influence.

A local police officer happened to be passing by. He knew Kimerly and her husband and was aware of Kim's Parkinson's disease. The officer attempted to explain the situation to the highway patrolman, but the patrolman insisted on giving Kimerly a ticket.

When it came time for Kim to appear in court for the case, she explained to the judge about her Parkinson's disease and her attempts to explain her condition to the patrolman.

The judge was appalled by the behavior of the patrolman and ordered him to make a full apology to Kimerly and to educate himself about Parkinson's disease.

The story shows that a great deal of education needs to be done about how Parkinson's disease affects people—not only with the general public but with those in public service positions, such as police, firefighters, and paramedics.

Tips for Safe Driving

○ Try to schedule errands for the time of day when you are feeling best.
○ Make the most of each trip. If you have more than one task you could complete in a trip, do so.
○ Avoid driving during rush hour or on heavily traveled routes when possible.
○ Don't drive long distances alone.

Be honest with yourself. If your medication is not working, or if you are tired, stiff, or experiencing a lot of tremors or dyskinesia, **don't drive**. Make other arrangements (wait awhile until you're feeling better; get someone else to drive; take a cab). Your life, and the lives of others, may depend upon your decision.

Since my diagnosis, I have traveled to Norway, Austria, and Italy, as well as across the United States. In fact, because of my PD-related activism, I have been to Miami, Phoenix, Philadelphia, Seattle, San Francisco, and Washington, DC. I have done most of these trips alone, and nearly all have gone very well. I only encountered difficulties while traveling when I didn't listen to my body and rest when I needed to do so. Having certain items with me on trips has made travel much easier.

Be prepared when you travel

While you need not travel like the Clampetts in the *Beverly Hillbillies* TV show, there are some things you shouldn't leave home without:

○ A list of all your current medications and dosages. If you want to be really high-tech, you can subscribe to Medic-Alert or a similar company. You purchase a stainless-steel bracelet or pendant with your name, ID number, and a phone number engraved on the back. You can also have a phrase, such as "Has Parkinson's disease," on the front. Paramedics or health professionals who contact the company will have access to the most recent medication and physician information that you have provided. Keep in mind, though, that this can be tricky to keep current if you are just starting a medication or trying different drugs such as antidepressants.

○ Contact information for your physician(s)

○ All of your medications, plus at least one full day's extra

○ Your health insurance contact information

○ Good comfortable walking shoes. (Ladies, try not to give in to the urge to put fashion before comfort or safety. As I write this, I am experiencing cramps in my left foot from wearing very lovely but highly impractical shoes at my brother's wedding. At least I had the good sense to remove them before dancing so that I didn't fall and break an ankle or wrist.)

○ A bottle of water for taking meds.

Useful travel items for overnight/out-of-town trips:

○ A telescoping (one that folds into itself) cane or walking stick. You never know when your medication may wear off unexpectedly or you may become tired from extra walking and need the extra support.

○ A medication timer or watch with an alarm. Even if you normally get by without one, using an alarm is helpful for keeping track of time zone changes and to avoid missing medications while on sightseeing tours or during a nice, long visit with an old friend.

Hotel tip:

○ Ask for handicapped-accessible rooms. Yes, I know that it is difficult to put aside one's pride the first time or two, but even if you don't need grab bars in your tub or shower at home, hotel and motel bathrooms can be very slippery. If an accessible room is not available, ask for a rubber bath mat to be placed in the tub.

Car travel tips:

○ Make frequent stretch stops. This will keep you from becoming even stiffer than you already are Stopping often is especially important if you are taking dopamine agonist medications, which have been shown to cause drowsiness.

○ Keep a large plastic bag in your glove box. If you find yourself having trouble sliding across leather/vinyl seats, easing the plastic under your bottom can provide just the slippery surface you need.

○ Keep a couple of extra doses of medication in your car (if you can keep them away from extreme heat), or in your wallet or purse.

○ When you're renting a car, choose a vehicle that is easy and comfortable to enter and exit. Although these vehicles are tougher on the environment and the pocketbook (because of their comparatively low gas mileage), sport-utility vehicles and minivans are generally just the right height.

Train travel tips:

○ On subways and commuter trains, where a high volume of passengers may cause standing-room-only conditions, take advantage of handicapped seating. Explain that you have Parkinson's disease, a condition that affects your balance, so you need to sit down. If anyone challenges your need for a seat, try using humor: "All right, I'll stand. . . . But you should know that I'm likely to end up in your lap if the train stops quickly!"

○ If you can't get a seat or choose to stand, be sure to hold tightly to a handrail.

○ Avoid traveling at peak times to minimize your stress about catching the train you need and getting a seat.

○ For all trains: arrive at the station or prepare for your stop early. Give yourself plenty of time to purchase your ticket or fare card and to get to the platform, and gather your belongings in preparation for disembarking (though avoid standing) before you pull in to the station.

○ Avoid walking while the train is moving whenever possible. If you need to go to the restroom or dining car, go slowly and hold on to handrails and seat backs for balance.

Air travel tips:

○ If you are unable to get the seat that you want when booking your flight online or with a travel agent, very often if you arrive at the airport a little early and check in at the ticket counter, the attendant can give you a bulkhead seat or an aisle seat toward the front of the plane. It doesn't hurt to ask. If that doesn't work, you can always ask the person in the seat you'd like if he is willing to switch seats with you.

○ Don't be shy about asking for assistance in getting through an airport. Many airports have electric carts that will transport you and your luggage to your gate. Others have wheelchairs available, with attendants to take you to the gate. Either of these options allows you to save your energy for your trip.

○ Take advantage of the opportunity to board the airplane first. It is much easier to get settled into your seat when you have ample room and fewer people standing in line behind you waiting for you to get your bag into the overhead bin. (I have always found a direct correlation between the number of people queuing up behind me and the difficulty I have doing things like stowing my bag or buckling my seatbelt.)

○ Have a great time, but pace yourself. Take naps. Sit down frequently. Drink plenty of fluids.

IN A SENTENCE:

Parkinson's disease will only make you homebound if you allow it to, but there are many commonsense steps to make you comfortable and keep you safe.

living

Sexuality and Intimacy

I SUSPECT that, given our society's schizophrenic approach to sex (scantily clad people in all media and sexual innuendo on TV and in advertising while at the same time there are debates over what to teach in sex ed in schools), research into PD's effects on sexuality and intimacy has not been a high priority. Unfortunately, we don't know much about how PD affects sex, but what we do know is that PD can have an adverse impact on our self-image, our interest in sex, and our physical capacity to enjoy it.

Medication and symptoms can get in the way

Unfortunately for men with PD, rigidity does not affect all parts of the body equally! (Sexuality is an awkward subject for Parkies, care partners, and health-care providers, so it helps to be able to laugh at ourselves.) The physical impacts of PD can cause impotence in men and may affect a woman's ability to achieve orgasm.

Tremors or muscle rigidity can make it awkward and embarrassing to find a position that is comfortable for more than a few seconds, and by the time you factor in fatigue, you may not have a whole lot of interest in sex. This can cause tension in your relationship, particularly if your partner's sex drive is stronger than yours.

Most of the SSRI antidepressants, anticholinergic drugs, and sedatives prescribed for PD can cause impotence and a decreased sex drive. Only you can decide if the sexual side effects are enough of a problem that you want to try a different medication. There are options available, so discuss the issue with your physician.

Plan ahead

If impotence or reduced sexual satisfaction has been a problem, talk to your doctor. She may be able to give you a prescription for Viagra or a similar drug. Viagra is helpful to many men, and to some women, too. Since you will need a prescription, you will have to do some planning. You must allow at least thirty minutes to more than an hour for drugs that treat erectile dysfunction (ED) to take effect. If you are a man with PD, you will need to factor in the timing of your Parkinson's medications so that they are not wearing off just as the ED medication kicks in. If you are a woman with PD and your partner takes ED medication, you will also need to consider the timing of your pills.

Make sure that the physician who prescribes Viagra is aware of other medications you may be taking.

Planning your sex life may seem a bit contrived, but doing so increases the likelihood that you will both enjoy yourselves. Schedule your "date" for a time of day when you are usually feeling your best. You can spend the time that it takes for the Viagra or similar drug to take effect by cuddling and holding each other.

Able but not interested

For most people, having a good sexual relationship is more than just physical attraction and hormones. We are looking for an emotional feeling of closeness as well. In other words, we're looking for intimacy.

Intimacy is defined as "a sense of belonging together; closeness." In most cases, that sense of belonging together is a primary reason for marrying or entering a committed relationship with someone. When we are intimately involved with someone, we can communicate our feelings and thoughts with a look or a particular phrase. At least, before PD we could.

PD can steal the subtlety and nuances of intimacy as muscle rigidity robs our faces of expression and our voices of inflection. Some of our most important tools of communication have been taken from us. And that is just what is happening inside of us. When you add the general chaos of daily life in many households, a dose of tremor or stiffness, a dash of guilt, and a sprinkling of resentment from your care partner, you have a recipe for an intimacy insecticide! Try recapturing the love bug by reading silly things together (like this paragraph), taking a moment to give your care partner a hug and say thank you for being there, or hiding love notes in your partner's wallet, purse, briefcase, or lunchbox.

Close relationships require more work

Keeping love alive is always a challenge, but the trials and tribulations of a chronic illness will really put you to the test. In most love relationships, you are able to come up with what is normal or typical for the two of you as a couple. Parkinson's is so variable and comprehensive in the ways it affects you that you never know quite what to expect. This is exhausting for both of you.

It is very common for people with Parkinson's to become frustrated with their life partner, because he or she doesn't understand what PD feels like. Instead of letting that come between you and your partner, try joining a support group. Support groups offer a great outlet where you can air your frustrations in front of people who do know what you're going through. They can validate your feelings and help you feel accepted and part of something larger.

Especially now, when you and your partner are still trying to figure out what this disease really is and how it will affect you, both of you are very vulnerable to the allure of someone who knows exactly what you are experiencing.

Having PD does not grant you an excuse to have an affair. If your emotional needs are not being met by your partner, now is a good time to talk about it. Parkinson's disease will either bring the two of you much closer together, or it will drive you apart if you let it.

I don't know of any successful long-term love relationship that is one-dimensional or based on only one shared interest. While a hobby, cause, or vocation may bring you together, your decision to be together presumably included other things that you have in common. Maintaining a connection to those other shared interests and experiences will keep your relationship dynamic and healthy.

It's a Date!

Nobody likes talking about all Parkinson's, all the time. Make a date with your partner to spend some time alone together. You may go to a movie; go out to dinner; go for a walk. But try working with this ground rule: no talk about PD. If one of you slips and brings up the forbidden subject, the other should stop the conversation with a kiss (or some other agreed-upon distraction).

Schedule these dates periodically when you are feeling particularly overwhelmed.

When the intimacy in your relationship is thriving, you will both be able to ask for what you need. Very often, that can mean just holding each other close or looking into each other's eyes. And if you are up for something more, you will feel comfortable telling or showing your partner what that is!

IN A SENTENCE:

Your PD symptoms, the physical and emotional toll on your care partner, medications, and other issues can affect your emotional and sexual relationship with your partner, and vice versa.

learning

Sleep

Many people in the early stages of Parkinson's disease are surprised to find that their sleep patterns have changed. The amount of time spent sleeping at night tends to be less than before, and you may find yourself feeling very tired during the day and in need of a nap. In fact, this is very common.

Getting enough rest is very important, whether it is all during "traditional" nighttime sleep hours or a combination of night sleep plus naps. Fatigue creates more stress, which can make your PD symptoms worse. It can also affect your immune system, making you more vulnerable to colds, viruses, and "whatever is going around." That is the last thing you need!

Two kinds of sleep problems

Sleep problems for people with PD fall into two main categories: staying asleep and staying awake. Remember though, as we get older, we typically need less sleep. So if you find yourself sleeping less than you did when you were younger, but otherwise feel rested and refreshed, you probably don't have a sleep problem.

Staying asleep

If you have difficulty falling asleep, wake frequently during the night, or are not remembering any dreams, there are several possible reasons for this.

Reduced sleep time or poor-quality sleep can be caused by PD symptoms. You may find yourself waking during the night due to muscle spasms or cramps. It may be difficult to turn to find a comfortable position. Muscle rigidity may affect your bladder, leading to the need to get up frequently during the night to urinate.

Restless legs syndrome is also common in people with Parkinson's. This means that your legs want to keep moving and you feel like you need to get up and walk around. There are medications that can help with this condition. (See page 11 for more information.)

For many people with Parkinson's, tremors cease while we are asleep. Others find that they are awakened from sleep by recurrence of tremors, because medication has worn off.

Anxiety also affects sleep. Some people find that they have difficulty falling asleep because their minds are reeling with all sorts of worries about what PD is doing to their lives. Others may be able to fall asleep without a problem, but if they are awakened for any reason, they have a tough time going back to sleep. I fall into this category. If I wake up during the night to use the bathroom or because of a cramp, my mind immediately starts creating a list of things I should be doing or forgot to do.

Medications can affect sleep, too. Most PD drugs bear labels warning that they may cause drowsiness, but everyone has different body chemistry. You may find that a drug causes insomnia. Sinemet and some of the antidepressant medications can cause nightmares or vivid dreams that may interrupt your sleep.

How to get more sleep

There are many measures that you can take to get more sleep and improve the quality of your sleep:

> Limit your caffeine intake. Too much caffeine, especially late in the day, can keep you awake at night. If you tend to drink a lot of coffee or tea, switch to decaffeinated varieties in the evening. Be on the lookout for caffeine lurking in unexpected places, such as some root beer and

orange soda varieties. (Those drinks are just empty calories anyway, but we all need treats now and then.)

Limit your alcohol intake. A glass of wine or beer can be a very relaxing, welcome accompaniment to dinner or at the end of a long day, but more is not better in this case. Having several drinks before bed may make you feel quite tired and help you to fall asleep, but the quality of the sleep you get will be poor. It will leave you feeling tired, dehydrated, and grumpy in the morning.

Another important reason to limit the amount of alcohol you drink is potential interaction with medications. Since many PD meds already induce drowsiness, alcohol can intensify that drowsiness and render you unfit to think clearly, drive, operate machinery, or do other complex tasks.

Exercise regularly—but not right before bed. Exercising daily or several times per week can help improve your sleep cycle. Just be sure not to exercise immediately before bed. Your adrenaline will be pumping and your muscles will be stimulated instead of relaxed, which will make it more difficult to fall asleep.

Have a place just for sleeping. Whether you sleep in a bed in your bedroom or a recliner in your den (it doesn't matter where you sleep or what you sleep on, as long as you're comfortable), your body will be more likely to let you sleep if you do not use that room or piece of furniture for many other things.

Don't eat a heavy meal just before bedtime. If you eat a large meal at 8:00 PM and go to bed at 9:00 PM, you will probably have heartburn or indigestion as well as insomnia. If you're feeling hungry before bed, have a small snack instead. Indeed, many people with PD—particularly older patients—have trouble taking in enough calories and need a snack.

Take a short nap. Napping during the day can reverse sleep cycles and can cause you to awaken more frequently during the night, so experiment with taking a short nap during the day. You may find that napping for fifteen to thirteen minutes, or even just resting quietly and focusing on your breathing during that time, will go a long way toward minimizing the amount of fatigue that you feel and help you be more alert during the day.

Try to keep to a schedule. This is sometimes easier said than done, but if you have raised any children, you know how much happier everyone is when the tykes are put to bed at a specific time and have a designated naptime. Adults are not so different.

Herbal/natural remedies. Warm milk really does contain a natural relaxing compound called tryptophan, so you may want to give that a try. Some people with Parkinson's report success with herbal remedies to help them sleep. Chamomile tea has long been touted for its relaxing properties. You may recall Beatrix Potter's tale about Peter Rabbit, whose mother served him chamomile tea after his stressful day in Mr. McGregor's garden. Valerian root is being studied by the National Center for Complementary and Alternative Medicine (NCCAM) as a sleep aid for people with PD. Do not use any herb or dietary supplements or OTC sleep remedies without first consulting your pharmacist. (I suggest talking with your pharmacist rather than solely relying upon your doctor's advice, because pharmacists are required to know about drug interactions and have access to many more resources about such things.)

If you have tried the options suggested above and are still having difficulty sleeping, talk to your doctor. He can offer additional suggestion and prescribe medications that can help.

Do You Like Sleep *Too* Much?

If you are a person who really loves to sleep, you want might to think about why it is that you enjoy it so much. Are you using it as a form of escape? This can be a sign of depression.

Staying awake

As I mentioned earlier, most PD medications come with colorful labels that warn, "May cause drowsiness. Alcohol may intensify this effect. Use care when operating a car or dangerous machinery." The sedative side effects can be welcome at night. However, during the day, when you need to stay awake to work or merely participate in the world around you, this drowsiness can be a problem. Joy, diagnosed at forty-six, tells of her experience with this problem:

> The most important fact, which I learned the hard way, was that some . . . of the drugs we take can make you extremely drowsy. I found this out when, on a bright, warm October day, I was behind the wheel of our car. Luckily, my husband was with me, because I fell asleep without realizing it! It was only when he screamed my name and grabbed the wheel that I became aware of what had happened.

Discuss daytime sleepiness with your doctor. You may be able to modify the dosage or timing of some of the medications you are taking.

Depression and anxiety can make you feel sleepy during the day. Review the depression inventory on page 77 to see if your drowsiness could be mood-related.

Daytime drowsiness can also be due to sleep apnea. Your doctor may order a sleep study to see if you have sleep apnea or some other physical condition that is affecting your sleep.

IN A SENTENCE:

Many people with PD have difficulties with sleep that may be due to muscle cramping, side effects of medication, urinary problems, or other issues.

Dealing with Your Employer

ALL OF the Parkies I know who are still working have been nervous about telling their employer. There seems to be a direct correlation between the level of anxiety about disclosing their PD and their need for the income, regardless of the economic sector in which they work.

Fear of others' reactions deters PD disclosure

Many newly diagnosed people with Parkinson's disease avoid telling their coworkers about their disease, because they believe that they will be treated differently and fear that they won't be treated as well as their coworkers. In retrospect, some of the Parkies I surveyed regretted their decision to delay or avoid telling their employers and coworkers about their illness.

> Make your employer aware that you have PD. The notification should be in writing. When you have to leave work, get disability from your employer. I didn't do either. I hid my PD from everyone. Why? I think I was embarrassed and I didn't want people treating me differently.
> —KEN, *diagnosed at age 52*

People's preconceived ideas about PD, or rather, about those who suffer from PD, surprised me. Specifically, I am in my third job since my diagnosis. I was honest with my employer at the time of my diagnosis. Almost immediately, I was relegated to a position where I would have almost no contact with guests. (I am a restaurant manager by profession.) At my second job, I was less than forthcoming about my situation, but when I told them about the Parkinson's disease, I was given verbal support. However, within two months, I was demoted and transferred twice. Each of the transfers was to a more physically demanding position. I can only guess that it would be easier for them if I quit [instead of their having to fire me]. I have been with my current company since February of 2003. After I started with them, I let them know about the PD. They have been extremely caring and supportive of my situation. I began having problems dealing with stairs about nine months ago. They moved me to a restaurant that was not only on one level, but also much closer to my home. I only wish I had found this company sooner than I did. —MARY, *diagnosed at 39*

Reasons to tell your employer

There are a number of reasons why you should tell your boss about your Parkinson's sooner rather than later. As is true with friends and loved ones, our bosses and fellow employees often notice more than we think they do when it comes to our Parkinson's disease. However, many of us who have had PD for several years have learned the hard way that PD is not usually the first problem employers suspect when they witness behaviors such as tremors, fatigue, and slurred speech.

One extremely compelling reason to tell your employer about your PD sooner rather than later is that if you make her aware of your condition before you receive a poor performance review or have the quality of your work questioned, the company is required to accommodate your disability. If you wait until you are called to the office because of a missed deadline or some performance issue, your boss may very well say, "You are just making excuses." This may seem unfair, but situations like this happen every day. It is your word against your employer's, and if you attempt to sue, chances are good that the company can afford more and better attorneys. Also, the fine print in many employment contracts makes you promise to settle any disputes through arbitration.

On the flip side, your boss could be a resource for information, ideas, contacts, and support. I was very lucky in that the staff at the nonprofit organization where I worked functions more like a family than a multilayered management bureaucracy. The management of the group went out of their way to accommodate my needs so that I could continue working as long as possible, yet also checked with me regularly to see if I felt overloaded.

Lastly, most of the people I surveyed found that their stress level—and their Parkinson's symptoms—subsided noticeably once they no longer had to keep their disease a secret.

Before you tell your employer

There are several things you should do before telling your employer. The most important is to decide whether you are simply going to inform your boss of your disease, or if you are also going to ask for some changes to be made that will allow you to keep working. You do not have to do both at the same time! In my case, I think it was a couple of years between the time I informed my employer of my diagnosis and my first request for some modifications to my position. (I did get voice-recognition software and a quieter workspace prior to my Parkinson's diagnosis.)

If you do not already know, check your company's personnel policy to see if it contains any information about sick leave and continuation of health benefits.

Check to see if your employer carries short-term or long-term disability insurance on you.

Talk with your doctor. She may be able to give you specific recommendations about how to maximize your work time. She may also be willing to write a letter of support. This is good ammunition to have when you talk to your boss about your work schedule, especially if it needs to change.

You may find it helpful to write out what you would like to say to your employer, or at least jot down the most important points that you want to be sure to cover. You might even want to do some role-playing with your care partner or someone you trust.

Talking to your boss

Talking to the boss is stressful for many people under the best of circumstances, so it is helpful to develop your game plan in advance. Here are some suggestions (this does not constitute legal advice) on how you might wish to proceed.

Make an appointment. You do not need to make the reason known when you schedule your time. If you have to book a specific amount of time, it is probably better to err on the side of having too much time and ending the meeting early than being in the middle of your request for accommodations and being told it will have to wait. Go in with a positive attitude. Assume that your employer will want to keep you. (That may not be the case, but if you go in expecting to have to hire a lawyer and take the case to court, you may create a self-fulfilling prophecy.) Emphasize your strong points, and be specific. Highlight the things you have done well, but don't exaggerate.

Ask for a written synopsis of your conversation and any proposals or decisions about accommodations that were discussed. This will help all parties remember what was said.

The Americans with Disabilities Act

The Americans with Disabilities Act (ADA) was passed by Congress in 1990 and took effect in 1992. The ADA is a federal law that was intended to prevent an employer from using a person's disability as a reason to avoid hiring him, to pay him lower wages, or to decline his promotion or deny his training.

The erratic nature of the symptoms of PD, particularly in the early years, can create some difficulties with employers, and the ADA can be helpful in gaining cooperation from your boss if other means have not worked.

Under the ADA, most employees are entitled to reasonable accommodations to allow them to keep their jobs. ("Reasonable accommodations" are defined in the ADA as "any modification or adjustment to a job or the work environment that will enable a qualified applicant or employee with a disability to participate in the application process or to perform essential job functions. Reasonable accommodation also includes adjustments to assure that a qualified individual with a disability has rights and privileges in employment equal to those of employees without disabilities."[1]) Some very small businesses may not be required to accommodate their staff, but many will. Accommodations do not have to be complicated or expensive.

Asking for workplace accommodations

When the time comes to ask for some changes to be made to your work, which may occur when you first tell your boss about your PD or years later, it is worthwhile to do some planning.

○ Don't start your conversation with a phrase like, "The ADA law says you have to accommodate me."
○ Have some ideas regarding accommodation. Even if you don't have exact technical fixes, you will be demonstrating consideration for your employer's position by saying, "I would like to try doing X differently for a week and then check in with you. Is that okay?"

Determining your accommodation needs

You will need to have some idea of the parts of your job that are becoming difficult. Here are some questions that will help you and your boss assess your needs and identify some options.

○ What are your symptoms? Which ones are currently having the most impact on your work?
○ Which tasks or parts of your job description are most affected, and in what ways?
○ Do you have any ideas for addressing these problems? Have you sought suggestions from others?
○ How do you plan to evaluate the usefulness of any accommodation that is made?

Accommodation Considerations for People with Parkinson's Disease

The Job Accommodation Network has already developed a fairly comprehensive list that I think will be helpful when you and your employer are discussing your needs. You may not be able to answer all of these questions right away, but they can serve as a place to begin.

Note: People with PD will develop some of these limitations and symptoms, but seldom develop all of them. Limitations will vary among individuals. Also note that not all people who have PD will need accommodations to perform their jobs, and many others may need only a few accommodations. The following is only a sample of the possibilities available. Numerous other accommodation solutions exist as well.

FINE MOTOR

- ◯ Implement ergonomic workstation design
- ◯ Provide arm supports
- ◯ Provide alternative computer access and keyguard
- ◯ Provide alternative telephone access
- ◯ Provide writing and grip aids
- ◯ Provide a page turner and a book holder
- ◯ Provide a note taker

GROSS MOTOR

- ◯ Reduce walking or provide a scooter or other mobility aid
- ◯ Provide parking close to the work site
- ◯ Provide an accessible entrance
- ◯ Install automatic door openers
- ◯ Provide an accessible route of travel to other work areas used by the employee
- ◯ Move workstation close to other work areas, office equipment, and break rooms

FATIGUE/WEAKNESS

- ○ Reduce or eliminate physical exertion and workplace stress
- ○ Schedule periodic rest breaks away from the workstation
- ○ Allow a flexible work schedule and flexible use of leave time
- ○ Allow work from home
- ○ Make sure materials and equipment are within reach range

SPEECH

- ○ Provide speech amplification, speech enhancement, or other communication device
- ○ Use written communication, such as e-mail or fax
- ○ Transfer to a position that does not require a lot of oral communication
- ○ Allow periodic rest breaks

MEDICAL TREATMENT ALLOWANCES

- ○ Provide flexible schedules
- ○ Provide flexible leave
- ○ Allow a self-paced workload with flexible hours
- ○ Allow employee to work from home
- ○ Provide part-time work schedules

DEPRESSION AND ANXIETY

- ○ Reduce distractions in work environment
- ○ Provide to-do lists and written instructions
- ○ Remind employee of important deadlines and meetings
- ○ Allow time off for counseling
- ○ Provide clear expectations of responsibilities and consequences
- ○ Provide sensitivity training to coworkers
- ○ Allow breaks to use stress management techniques
- ○ Develop strategies to deal with work problems before they arise
- ○ Allow telephone calls during work hours to doctors and others for support
- ○ Provide information on counseling and employee assistance programs

COGNITIVE IMPAIRMENT

- ○ Provide written job instructions when possible
- ○ Prioritize job assignments
- ○ Allow flexible work hours
- ○ Allow periodic rest breaks to reorient
- ○ Provide memory aids, such as schedulers or organizers
- ○ Minimize distractions
- ○ Allow a self-paced workload
- ○ Reduce job stress
- ○ Provide more structure

ACTIVITIES OF DAILY LIVING

- ○ Allow use of a personal attendant at work
- ○ Allow use of a service animal at work
- ○ Make sure the facility is accessible
- ○ Move workstation closer to the restroom
- ○ Allow longer breaks
- ○ Refer to appropriate community services

Reprinted from the Job Accommodation Network Web site, www.jan.wvu.edu. The Job Accommodation Network is a service of U.S. Department of Labor's Office of Disability Employment Policy.

Telling coworkers

Disclosing your disease to your boss is not the same as telling your coworkers. There is no compelling legal reason to tell them. You may choose to tell some, but not all, of the people you work with. You can base your decision on how much you interact with a person, whether you trust him to keep the information in confidence, and so on.

IN A SENTENCE:

> There are many things to keep in mind when considering whether and how to let your boss know that you have Parkinson's disease, and the Americans with Disabilities Act (ADA) offers job protection for most people.

learning

Dealing with Dementia

A CERTAIN percentage of people with Parkinson's disease—
I found statistics that varied from 15 percent to 25 percent all
the way up to 80 percent—will develop dementia. For many of
us with PD, this is the potential effect that we fear most.

What is dementia?

Dementia is a brain disease that affects a person's memory,
thinking, speech, and movement. Forgetfulness is one of the first
signs of dementia, so when we Parkies forget where we put our
car keys, or our reason for going from one room to another, we
often panic and assume we are developing dementia.[2]

Not everyone who has PD develops dementia

The good news is not everyone who has PD will develop
dementia. However, I can't tell you what your chances are for getting it. Finding consistent statistics on dementia in PD rates is
more complicated than getting estimates of PD cases. This is due
to misdiagnosis, differences in the definition of dementia, and
the way this type of information is collected.

One study that placed the overall rate of PD in the community at 99.4 cases per 100,000 determined the dementia rate in people with PD to be 41.3 percent. The likelihood of dementia increases with age (12.4 percent in people of age fifty to fifty-nine, rising to 68.7 percent in patients over eighty).[3]

Dementia is very rare in people with Parkinson's who were diagnosed before age fifty, even if you have PD for a long time. Conversely, people who are diagnosed with PD after age seventy are much more likely to develop dementia.

Risk factors for dementia

The following factors make it more likely that you will develop dementia:

○ You're male.
○ You are over age seventy.
○ Your primary PD symptoms are slowness of movement and balance/walking difficulties.
○ You have a history of depression.
○ You scored around 25 (moderate impairment) on the Universal Parkinson's Disease Rating Scale (UPDRS). There is a copy of the UPDRS in Resources.
○ You have experienced symptoms of mania or psychosis, or become manic or agitated while taking Sinemet.
○ You have facial masking (little or no facial expression).
○ You come from a low-income background without much formal education.

Symptoms of dementia

Dementia involves more than just forgetting things occasionally. There are a number of signs that would have to be present for your doctor to suspect dementia.

○ forgetfulness
○ problems retrieving memories without the assistance of a cue or clue
○ difficulty concentrating or paying attention

○ difficulty planning or making decisions (these are often referred to as "executive function")
○ slowed thinking
○ lack of motivation; apathy
○ poor judgment
○ difficulty processing and understanding visual information[4]

It can be difficult to discern the difference between the type of dementia found in people with Alzheimer's disease versus that in PD or another condition called *dementia with Lewy bodies* (DLB). Lewy bodies are present in individuals with each of the three conditions, so it is likely that there is some relationship.

Regardless of the age of the person with PD, dementia does not generally occur early in the disease. Developing Parkinson-like motor symptoms at the same time as those of dementia usually signals another condition.

It may not be dementia

There are other causes of dementia symptoms that should be investigated as well. For example, many of the symptoms listed above also apply to depression. Some individual medications can induce symptoms that resemble dementia, or two or more drugs may react to create dementia symptoms. Other conditions that may mimic some symptoms of dementia include nutritional deficiencies (e.g., B_{12}); hypoglycemia; infections such as meningitis; Alzheimer's disease or other brain-related conditions unrelated to PD; and even dehydration![5]

So if you or your care partner have concerns about any cognitive changes that you have noticed, let your doctor know right away—but don't automatically fear the worst.

Treatment for dementia

Unfortunately, there is no cure for dementia, but there are ways to control the symptoms. Anticholinergic drugs and medications used to treat Alzheimer's disease may help for a while. Because dementia is so bewildering and frightening for people with the condition, and, for their partners, they may focus all of their energy on trying to address the dementia symptoms. Parkinson's does not go away with the onset of dementia. PD symptoms need to continue to be treated, while adding medications to treat depression or other mood disorders or psychoses.

IN A SENTENCE:

> Dementia occurs in some Parkinson's patients, and the symptoms resemble those of Alzheimer's disease.

MONTH **10**

Planning Your Financial Future

WHEN I was diagnosed with Parkinson's disease, I was in my early thirties. At that time, I wasn't even saving for retirement at the hale and hearty age of sixty-five. I certainly was not prepared to have to retire at forty! Of course, many cases of PD are diagnosed much later, and it is very likely that you have put more foresight and planning into your retirement years than I have. But in my chats with other people with Parkinson's, most have expressed surprise at the insidious impacts that this disease has on every aspect of their budget. Below I've identified common categories of costs that you can incur as a result of PD. Most are obvious, but you may not have thought of them as a package deal.

Medications

Every health plan with which I am familiar seems to require a co-payment for most prescriptions. Even if your co-pay is five dollars per thirty-day supply of a medication, keep in mind that you will be on some of these medications for a number of years. At some point, you may be on multiple medications for PD, and possibly other conditions as well.

Mounting out-of-pocket drug costs has been an issue of

concern with seniors for many years. You may be able to save some money by getting your medications filled online or through mail order. With those methods, you will need to be sure that you are dealing with a reputable company. Some insurance programs have a mail-order company with whom they have a contract. If you are shopping online, look for a company that is a member of the Better Business Bureau. This doesn't mean you will never have a problem, but you know that they take customer feedback seriously.

If your current financial plan does not include a line item for medications, add one now. If you are not currently taking medication for your PD but can afford to put some extra money aside, it would allow you to be better prepared to deal with expensive drugs that may come later. (For instance, my copayment for my Mirapex prescription is $24/month. That is almost $300/year for just one medication.)

Complementary therapies

Some of the complementary therapies for PD may be covered by your insurance provider—physical therapy, for example—but many are not. If you have found that a weekly massage greatly reduces your stiffness, it would be worthwhile to see if that treatment can be fit into your budget somehow.

Nutritional supplements are generally not covered by health insurance and can be quite expensive. However, you may decide that you want to take an antioxidant supplement to reduce the impact of free radicals on your brain. Or take a calcium supplement to help keep your bones strong. These are choices that you and your health practitioner should discuss. Spending ten dollars per month on vitamins does not seem like much, but when factored in with all of the other financial costs of PD, it may become significant.

Assistive devices

There are literally thousands of devices and products aimed at making your life easier. Walkers and scooters are often covered by health insurance or Medicare, but not always. If you find yourself in need of a walker or scooter and your insurance won't cover it, that's a big expense you'll need to find a way to absorb. Smaller items, such as long-handled shoehorns, voice-recognition software, and handrails for stairs, are unlikely to be covered. Some of these tools could literally save your life but do require a small investment.

Hired help

If you hate housework (as I do) and can afford to pay someone to come in on a weekly or biweekly basis, consider adding this line item to your financial plan. It could reduce your stress and risk of injury and allow you to make the most of your free time.

Transportation

Last spring, I mentioned to my husband that I had begun to have difficulty getting in and out of my station wagon. I said this just before the auto show. Paul goes to the show every year, and it is a way for him to have some free time with friends. Last year, however, I had to go, too, to check different vehicles for their seat height and adjustability and other features.

You don't need to purchase a brand-new vehicle, but there may come a time that you will buy a different one that is more accessible.

You might also choose to take cabs or hire a driver. Some communities offer public transportation vehicles that can be summoned by phone to take handicapped individuals to specific destinations. There are a number of options if PD impairs your ability to drive. It is a good idea to start thinking now about how you would like to handle the likelihood that at some point your mobility will be impaired.

Housing

When we bought our first home in 1995, we had planned to stay in it indefinitely. It was a 1910 Dutch Colonial with hardwood floors, a built-in buffet, ornately carved woodwork, and lots of windows. At the time, we didn't mind that all three bedrooms and the only bathroom were upstairs, or that the laundry was in the basement, or that the doorways were narrow. But these features were very apparent to the occupational therapist and physical therapist who visited our home in 2001.

We learned very quickly that most of the homes on the market that were in our price range were not accessible either. Shopping for a home the second time around was very different. We now had to look at the width of the doorways— could they accommodate a walker or a wheelchair? Was there room to move about in the bathroom with a walker or wheelchair? Was the bathroom large enough to someday hold a roll-in shower? Such a modification requires a lot of space and is expensive. It means tiling a large enough area of the floor and walls to allow someone who uses a walker or wheelchair to roll in under the showerhead—rather like the way locker rooms are designed.

If you are very lucky, the place in which you live will require little or no modification as your PD progresses. For the majority of us, the progression of our disease will mean significant remodeling or moving to a new place altogether.

This was a big issue, and one that we had not considered when I was diagnosed. I urge you to have your home or apartment evaluated now, as early in your disease as possible. That will maximize the time you have to think about what you might have to fix or where you want to move. Discussing this now will give you much greater flexibility than waiting until you fall and break your hip and are forced to spend weeks recuperating in a nursing home because your house is not accessible.

Travel

If you are retired and enjoy spending winters in warm climates or driving your RV across the country, you do not have to stop because of PD. But you may have to modify your mode of transportation or your accommodations as your disease progresses, and this will cost money. For example, if you like to camp and would normally sleep in a tent, the rigidity and stiffness of Parkinson's might mean that you would be more comfortable sleeping in a trailer or RV.

If you are still working and had planned on traveling after you retired, I would urge you to reconsider. Seize the moment if you can work it into your budget. You will be able to do much more now.

If you don't already have a financial adviser, now would be a good time to find one. Try to find someone who has some experience dealing with clients with a chronic illness. (It may be tough to find one who is well-versed in Parkinson's disease.) Good planning now can make your life with PD much more enjoyable.

IN A SENTENCE:

> *Living with PD is expensive, so financial planning now will help you and your family to have a financially secure future later.*

learning

Surgery to Treat PD Symptoms

BEFORE LEVODOPA was discovered, surgery was a common treatment for PD. When Sinemet became available in the 1960s, it began a period of drug therapy as the primary means for dealing with PD. In the late twentieth century, as side effects of Sinemet got more attention and new surgical techniques were developed, surgery became more popular again.

Surgery may be an option much later in your disease

Many people with Parkinson's disease reach a point after several years when medications are no longer controlling the disease to their satisfaction. At that point you may begin to think about surgical options and bring up the topic during a doctor visit, or your health-care provider may suggest surgery as an option. Surgery is not a treatment offered to those who are newly diagnosed.

Surgery is not a cure

Just as medications, exercise, massage, and other therapies treat the symptoms of PD but do not make it go away, surgery can only offer temporary relief—it is not a cure. Many people with Parkinson's who have surgery report years of reduction of physical symptoms.

There are different types of surgery

There are several types of surgery performed to treat PD, and your doctor will discuss them with you in the context of your symptoms.

Success rates

PEOPLE ALWAYS want to know what the success rates are for various procedures. It is a fair question, but one that is tough to answer.

"Success" is a relative term that will depend upon the type of symptoms you have, their severity, your overall health, and the quality of the brain imaging done prior to surgery, any side effects that result from the surgery, and the skill and experience of your surgeon. The interpretation of all of these factors is very subjective. For example, if a pallidotomy virtually eliminated your tremors but made your speech unintelligible, would you consider it a success? A failure? Both?

If you reach a point in your disease that you are contemplating surgery, your doctors should discuss what your expectations are and be able to give you some indications as to whether those expectations are reasonable.

ABLATIVE SURGERY

Some surgical procedures work by destroying an area of the brain that is too active. Such operations are called **ablative surgery**, or **lesioning surgery**. The destroyed area is called a **lesion**.

These types of surgeries are nearly always performed on only one side **(unilateral)** of the brain. The right side of our brain controls functions on the left side of the body, and vice versa, so any operation would be done on the side opposite of the one on which you experience most of your symptoms. **Bilateral** (both sides of the brain) procedures pose a significant risk for severe speech and swallowing impediments after the surgery.[1]

PALLIDOTOMY

This procedure has been in use for about fifty years. It involves the destruction of part of the *globus pallidus*. By eliminating an area where there is too much communication or "cross-talk" between the neurons in that region, the pallidotomy reduces tremors, rigidity, slowed movements, and dyskinesia in some patients. There is some debate in the scientific community as to how long these effects last, but this seems to be true of any treatment for PD, regardless of whether it is drug therapy, surgery, or some other intervention.

There are a number of potential side effects associated with the procedure. About 11 percent of people who have a pallidotomy have at least partial vision loss.[2] Other effects can include cognitive impairment and increased risk of brain hemorrhage (bleeding in the brain) or stroke.

THALAMOTOMY

A thalamotomy involves making a lesion in a part of the brain called the **thalamus**. This procedure is very rarely performed on people with Parkinson's these days, because while it is very effective for tremor, it does not help with rigidity or slowed movements. This surgery is still used for people with essential tremor.

Potential complications of this surgery can include weakness or numbness on the side opposite the surgery; impaired vision; seizures; difficulty walking; and slurred speech. These effects, when they occur, are not always permanent.[3]

DBS

A new type of brain surgery for PD called **deep-brain stimulation (DBS)** was invented in the late 1980s.[4] It involves placing a thin metal electrode that is about the size of a piece of spaghetti in the thalamus, a portion of the globus pallidus called the **globus pallidus interna (GPi),** or a third area of the brain called the **subthalamic nucleus (STN),** depending on the symptoms you hope to affect.

The electrode is hooked up to a battery pack that is inserted into the person's chest. The battery powers the electrode, allowing it to provide electrical stimulation at a frequency of 100 to 180 hertz. The battery can be turned on and off with a magnet that you wave over the spot in your chest where it was implanted, so when you're feeling good you can save the battery by turning it off, and then you can switch it back on when your symptoms begin to bother you. Saving the battery is important, because when it runs out of juice, you have to have it surgically removed and a new one implanted. The lifetime of the battery varies from person to person.

Because the electrodes, also called stimulators, can be moved, switched off, or removed and the frequency adjusted, bilateral surgery is common.[5] The technology has now advanced to the point that stimulators can be put into two regions instead of just one. This can be very helpful, since many people with Parkinson's who opt for DBS surgery have experienced progression of their PD such that they have symptoms on both sides of their body.

DBS Is Tailored to Individual Needs

With DBS, the symptoms you want to treat dictate where the surgeon puts the electrode(s). For example, placing them in the thalamus will significantly reduce tremor. When the electrodes are placed in the GPi or STN regions, tremor, rigidity, slowed movements, and difficulty walking can all be improved. Dyskinesia can also be significantly reduced and people with Parkinson's can usually take much less medication.[6]

The stimulators are programmed and adjusted or tuned by health professionals who have been specially trained. Periodically, you will go in for additional programming or tuning in response to changes in your symptoms.

Complications Can Occur

Bleeding in the brain can lead to a stroke and occurs in approximately 2 percent of patients. Infection occurs in about 4 percent of patients.[7] The infections can be treated but may require the removal of the entire system.

Health Insurance Usually Covers DBS

DBS surgery of the thalamus, Gpi, and STN were approved by the Food and Drug Administration for treatment of PD in 1997, 2002, and 2002, respectively.[8] Medicare will now pay for DBS, as will many private insurers. Check with your individual insurance provider before scheduling the procedure to see if the operation is covered and at what level.

If you are contemplating surgery

While many people do benefit from the various types of brain surgery used to treat Parkinson's disease, there are some key points to consider, because it is not for everyone.

○ Different surgical procedures target specific symptoms, so a procedure that helps one of your friends with her symptoms might not be appropriate for yours.

○ DBS is expensive! Pallidotomies and thalamotomies are rare enough that I couldn't find cost figures. I know a couple of Parkies who had DBS surgery before it was given FDA approval as a treatment. At that time, they reported estimates of $60,000 to $80,000 for the procedure, and they had to petition their insurance companies to pay for it. Medtronic, the company that makes the Activa® DBS system, reported an estimate of $50,000 to $60,000 in May 2004.[9] That figure includes the system components, the doctors' fees, and the hospital stay.

○ As with any surgical procedure, there is risk involved. You must be sure you can live with the potential consequences of the surgery.

○ Emerging research indicates DBS may worsen preexisting psychiatric conditions such as depression, anxiety, and drug addiction. Some patients have become hypersexual, apathetic, or aggressive after surgery. Others have begun gambling.[10]

DBS-STN.org, a new group that is affiliated with the Parkinson's Alliance, is collecting information to study these potential side effects of DBS and to improve the quality of life of DBS patients. You can visit the Web site or call 1–800–579–8440.

Medical technology is evolving at an incredible rate, so make sure that your doctor keeps you updated. If and when you consider surgery, the landscape will almost certainly have changed considerably. Surgery has helped many people with PD to lead longer, fuller lives.

IN A SENTENCE:

> *Several surgical treatments are being used to treat, but not cure, many PD symptoms, including tremors, rigidity, and dyskinesia.*

Insurance and PD

THERE ARE many forms of insurance in our world today, and nearly all of them can have some sort of impact on you and your family if you have Parkinson's disease.

Stay on top of the paperwork

It is very easy to become overwhelmed in a sea of forms and receipts as you deal with more doctors and more prescriptions. It's important to keep ahead of the bills and make sure insurance claims get submitted. You and your partner will probably want to have frequent check-ins about the status of the paperwork and have someone designated to deal with it. If you assume that "one of us will get around to it sometime," you could lose a great deal of money as well as your credit rating.

Information on insurance products

I am deeply indebted to my friend and fellow Parkie, Jack Hungelmann, for the information that he provided from articles he has written and from his excellent resource book, *Insurance for Dummies*.[1] Jack has been in the insurance business for thirty years and has had PD for eight. This combination puts him in a unique position to give us advice.

What follows is a general overview of the major types of insurance and some of their good points and bad points relative to PD. Your individual policies or coverage may vary.

Taking the time now to evaluate the status of your insurance coverage can potentially save you a great deal of money, time, and hassle in years to come.

IN A SENTENCE:

> *Whether you have health insurance, life insurance, and other insurance products can have a very big impact on your financial future.*

Insurance Programs and Their Financial Implications for People with PD

Insurance Product	Paid by	Positive aspects	Negative aspects
Group health insurance	At least partially funded by employer	• *Usually* offered to new employees without exclusion (preexisting conditions covered)	• Stops when you stop working for that employer
Individual health insurance	You	• Can be covered until age 65 without cancellation or price increase • Can cover spouse and kids	• Have to prove that you are healthy to qualify • Your application could be denied because of your PD • Coverage of PD expenses could be excluded
Group long-term disability	Employer	• Offered to new employees without exclusion • Payable until 65 if you become disabled • *May* allow you to convert to individual policy if you leave the position	• May have to have coverage for 12 to 24 months before PD-related disability would be covered • Benefits are about 45% of salary (60% of salary minus taxes withheld) • No cost-of-living adjustment • Don't usually have partial benefit (can't work part-time and have insurance make up the rest of your salary)
Individual long-term disability	You	• Can be kept until 65 even if you change jobs • May be renewable at locked price at 65 • No taxes withheld because you paid with after-tax funds • Can collect benefits from other sources without decrease in this policy disbursement • May have partial disability option	• Proof of good health is required to qualify

Insurance Product	Paid by	Positive aspects	Negative aspects
Group life insurance	Employers pay for base amount; you can pay for additional coverage	• Free coverage–why not?! • Employer-paid portion may be able to be converted to permanent coverage (which will be more expensive, but having PD, take what you can get)	• Additional individual coverage is probably cheaper on the open market • Free coverage usually stops when you leave the job
Individual life insurance	You	• Term insurance is cheaper and a good bet for covering families with young kids • Permanent insurance more suited to covering a care partner who is or will have to be caring for PWP–buy enough coverage to replace income and hire caregiver for you	• Proof of good health is required to qualify
Long-term care insurance	You	• Covers hired help with daily personal care activities • Look for a policy that will cover benefits anywhere (assisted living, hospice, nursing home, in-home)	• Too late for people with Parkinson's (PWP) if you don't already have coverage, but get a policy for your care partner
Medicare supplement insurance	You	• A good policy will cover hospitalization for up to one year beyond Medicare allowance; travel outside the U.S. and Canada; pays up to 80% of doctor bills over Medicare allowance	
Consolidated Omnibus Budget Reconciliation Act (COBRA)	You	• Allows you to continue your group health insurance policy for up to 18 months after leaving a position	• Tends to be expensive

Insurance Product	Paid by	Positive aspects	Negative aspects
Health Insurance Portability and Accountability Act (HIPAA)	You	• Guarantees portability of health insurance to age 65 • You *cannot be excluded* for having PD or any other preexisting condition	• Individual states determine insurance provider
State health insurance pools	You	• Your state may have a state-run plan for people who cannot qualify with private insurers • Rates typically 20% above that charged for someone with no health problems (if you consider the fact that you cannot qualify for other insurance, 20% isn't all that bad)	• Your state may not offer such a program (check with your state's insurance department)
Health Savings Account (HSA)	You	• "Allows people who buy private health insurance the opportunity to save a significant amount on health insurance costs (30 to 50 percent) by purchasing a government-approved high deductible health plan (HDHP) and then prefunding up to 100 percent of the deductible each year in a savings account where the contributions are 100 percent tax deductible (much like an IRA contribution)." • Healthy care partners can save a lot of money	• Lots of paperwork • PWP likely to meet or exceed deductibles may not be worth it for us
Social Security disability benefits	Federal government	• If your disability has lasted or is expected to last at least 12 months and you have been disabled (not working) for 5 months, you may qualify • Regardless of your age, after two years of Social Security disability benefits, you automatically qualify for Medicare and for the right to buy the best Medicare supplement you can find	• PWP are often denied on their first application because of the way Social Security defines ability to work (you may not be able to do your job, but if SS thinks that there are some jobs that you could physically do, your claim may be turned down)

Insurance Product	Paid by	Positive aspects	Negative aspects
Medicare	Federal government	• No exclusions for preexisting conditions	• Must be 65 years or older or have been collecting Social Scurity disability benefits for 2 years • No coverage outside the U.S. and Canada • You are responsible for charges Medicare won't pay • A 90-day limit on hospitalization (60 bonus days allowed once)
Medicaid	Federal government	• Coverage of last resort	• Can only qualify if your income is at or below the poverty level and you have no assets (e.g., if you own your home, you would not qualify, because that is a substantial asset)

Source: Hungelmann, "What Young-Onset Persons with Parkinson's Need to Know about Insurance."

learning

Help to Find a Cure

ONE OF the first questions I found myself asking when I was diagnosed with PD—right after "Why me?" and "What caused this?"—was, "What is being done to find a cure?" I learned that a lot of research is being done to answer this question and that I can be part of these efforts by participating in **clinical trials**. These can be research projects that help scientists to learn about various aspects of a disease or they can be studies to evaluate new medications, treatments, or procedures. All play important roles in finding the cause(s) and cure for Parkinson's disease.

Parkinson's disease is considered to be a "gateway" disease, one for which research provides information that may open the door to treating/curing other diseases.

Clinical trials funded with federal dollars are often held at the National Institutes of Health (NIH) facilities in Bethesda, Maryland, or at universities or federally funded research centers that apply for government grants for such research. These studies may be what is called basic, or "bench," research that informs the overall knowledge about a number of diseases, or they may be specific to Parkinson's disease.

PDTrials.org = One-Stop Shopping

PDTRIALS.ORG IS a new collaborative effort by the American Parkinson's Disease Association (APDA), Michael J. Fox Foundation (MJF), National Institutes of Health (NIH), National Parkinson Foundation (NPF), Parkinson's Action Network (PAN), Parkinson's Alliance, Parkinson's Disease Foundation (PDF), and WEMOVE (Worldwide Education and Awareness for Movement Disorders). The organization aims to include all of the PD-related clinical trials going on at any one time in the United States. This ambitious project was launched in 2005 and has information about federally funded research projects being done by NIH and other agencies, as well as private trials being conducted by pharmaceutical companies, medical device manufacturers, or other private entities.

PDTrials.org is advised by two PD-advocacy groups: the Parkinson's Pipeline Project and the Parkinson's Study Group.

You can check out this wonderful new resource online at www.pdtrials.org or by e-mailing info@pdtrials.org. If you do not have access to a computer or prefer to receive printed information, call the Advancing Parkinson's Therapies information request line at 1–888–823–8889.

Types of clinical trials

The clinical trials that help researchers to learn more about specific aspects of PD or other illnesses do not treat your disease. Instead, you may be asked to perform tasks, such as recalling a series of words or doing repetitive motions. Or you may have blood, urine, spinal fluid, or other samples tested to see if your body has something in it that people without PD do not have, or if you are lacking something—an enzyme, a gene, a chemical—that people without PD have.

Drug or device studies may be conducted by government agencies, universities, participating hospitals, and clinics or facilities operated by pharmaceutical manufacturers or medical device manufacturers.

The drugs or medical devices being tested for these studies can fall into several categories:

○ The drug or device has been approved by the Food and Drug Administration for human use, but not for treating Parkinson's disease.

○ The drug or device has gone through enough stages of testing in cell cultures and animal models to allow testing on humans, but you are part of a group that will be among the first people to try the drug or device.

○ These types of studies are usually "double-blind." That means that they are set up in such a way that during the study, neither you nor your health-care providers know whether you are receiving the research drug or a **placebo**. After the study period is over, you learn whether or not you were actually receiving the drug. In the case of medical devices being tested, double blind studies may involve "sham surgery." This means that you do undergo surgery and you do have some sort of device implanted, but it is not functional.

○ The drug or device has been through many levels of testing and you know for certain that you will be receiving the medication or the device. These research projects are called "open-label" studies, because everyone involved—you, your care partner, your health-care provider, and the drug or device maker—all know that you are receiving the product being tested. You would be monitored to see whether or not it helped any of your symptoms. You should also be asked about and monitored for side effects or unintended consequences of the drug or device.

Basic information about clinical trials

Your transportation to and from the study site is almost always subsidized or completely covered by the testing entity. If you participate in a study in your own community, you may be reimbursed for mileage, tolls, and parking that are necessary expenditures to ensure your participation.

If you need to stay overnight because of the travel distance or length of the study, accommodations are generally provided. Many studies also budget for an allowance for meals and other expenses associated with travel.

In addition to providing travel and accommodations, some studies also pay you a fee for your participation.

Depending on the drug's stage in the FDA approval process, you may be allowed to continue on the medication if you were receiving it during the study, or offered a chance to try it if you were in the placebo group.

This can be one frustrating aspect of clinical trials. You may take part in a study from which you see positive results. Maybe your tremors subside, or you can walk more easily or think more clearly. However, at the end of the study, the drug may need to go through one or more additional phases before it is available for your use.

NET-PD: Clinical Trials for Neuroprotection

THE NINDS has begun recruiting volunteers for a project called Neuroprotection Exploratory Trials in Parkinson's Disease, or NET-PD. Drugs or chemical compounds in this study are being tested for their ability to stave off the progression of PD.

If you are interested in learning more about this research and potential participation, send an e-mail to info@parkinsontrial.org or call 1–800–352–9424. You can also visit the project's Web site at parkinsontrial.org/netpd-drugs.htm/.

IN A SENTENCE:

> *Clinical trials are research studies used to help determine the cause of a disease, the effectiveness of therapies, and potential cures; and you and your family may be eligible to participate.*

living

What You Can Do to Raise Awareness of PD

IN MANY ways, just getting out of bed in the morning and going out into the world to interact with others is raising awareness about Parkinson's disease. This helps educate people about PD symptoms and demonstrates that your disease does not define who you are.

But you can do even more to raise awareness about Parkinson's disease by participating in events like walkathons or golf tournaments organized by local or national PD groups. To learn more about which national organizations may have groups or chapters in your area, consult the Resources section of this book.

Political advocacy

The first time I heard it, I felt a kinship with the quote by Maggie Kuhn of the Gray Panthers, "Speak out, even though your voice shakes." At the time, it had meaning for me because my voice would quaver with nervousness when I testified at public hearings or speak at rallies on environmental issues. Now, PD has given it an even deeper meaning. Although my voice—and my body—shake, I refuse to let those little details get in the way of speaking up when something is important to me. Yes, I get embarrassed, and yes, I know that many people are uncomfortable watching me struggle to get the words out. But that discomfort can be the impetus for change.

The *American Heritage Dictionary* defines advocacy as "the act of pleading or arguing in favor of something such as a cause, idea, or policy; active support." In other words, speaking up for what you believe or "walking your talk."

On a political level, Parkinson's advocacy means communicating with people—especially policy makers—about stem cell research, funding for the National Institutes of Health (NIH), and other issues that can affect the support, treatment, and cure for people with Parkinson's disease and their families.

Exercising your advocacy does not have to be time-consuming, difficult, or stressful. There are a number of simple things that you can do:

○ Write a letter to the editor of your neighborhood or community newspaper about a Parkinson's-related issue, such as how your life has been affected by the high cost of prescription drugs, or the lack of widely available accessible housing. You don't need to be an expert. Just pick something that you feel passionate about and write about that. Refer to experiences in your own life to make the topic real for people.

○ Check with the newspaper first to see how many words they will accept, how to submit your letter, and so on.

○ Call, fax, e-mail, or visit your state and federal legislators about an issue or issues that are important to you. (Note: If you're trying to reach a member of Congress, writing a letter and sending it via postal mail is definitely not a timely way to communicate. Mail going to Capitol Hill goes through extensive processing, including irradiation. If you do not have access to e-mail, you could ask your child or grandchild to do it for you.)

○ Call in to make a comment when you're listening to talk radio programs on PD-related topics such as the cost of prescription drugs, mental health, disability, supplemental Social Security, and stem cells.

○ Talk to your family friends, neighbors, and coworkers about how Parkinson's disease has affected your life.

You do not have to be an expert to talk with your representatives in the state legislature or in Congress. It is important that you form your own opinion. If an issue seems too complex and you don't feel comfortable expressing an opinion, that is fine. But remember that part of advocacy is educating others about PD, and you are an expert in how it affects you, whether you want to be or not!

Just being out in public is a way of raising awareness about PD, especially if you are willing to be open about it. (After a while, it will probably become obvious. If I notice someone looking at me strangely, I will explain, "I have Parkinson's disease. That's why I am [shaky, wiggly, stiff]." If you can have a sense of humor about it, it makes things easier for everyone.)

You can also choose to be active in local Parkinson's groups or participate in local or national Parkinson's events. One such event is the Unity Walk, sponsored by all of the national PD groups. It is held annually in April (Parkinson's Disease Awareness Month) in New York's Central Park. The Unity Walk is a wonderful way to raise money for Parkinson's disease research, raise awareness, make new friends, and get great information.

PARKINSON'S ACTION NETWORK (PAN) is the "unified education and advocacy voice of the Parkinson's community, fighting to ease the burden and find a cure." This Washington, DC–based organization has volunteers in more than thirty-seven states who keep others apprised of the status of federal funding and policies that affect the Parkinson's disease community. Anyone can be part of PAN. You do not need to have PD or be a care partner for someone who does. All are welcome.

To find out more about PAN and see whether there are advocates in your state that you can contact, visit their Web site, www.parkinsonsaction.org, or call 1–202–638–4101 or 1–800–850–4726.

IN A SENTENCE:

> *Every day, you have an opportunity to teach others about Parkinson's disease as you go about your daily life, but there are ways to maximize that influence.*

learning

Emerging Therapies for Parkinson's Disease

THERE ARE scientists all over the United States and the world working on ways to halt the progression of PD, cope with the symptoms of the disease, and repair the damage that the disease causes in the brain. None of these ventures has produced a cure yet, but we will still reap great benefits from this important work.

Promising drug therapies

Research into new drug therapies for the treatment of Parkinson's disease falls into two categories: the development of new drugs or "novel compounds," and identification of new uses of drugs that are already on the market.

NOVEL COMPOUNDS

Substances that are believed to protect your substantia nigra—that part of the brain that makes dopamine—from harm, or at least forestall further damage, are called "neuroprotective agents." The National Institutes of Health (NIH) has convened the Committee to Identify Neuroprotective Agents in Parkinson's

(CINAPS) to review information on drugs or other compounds that may have neuroprotective benefits. The committee, supported by the National Institute of Neurologic Disorders and Stroke (NINDS), has identified a dozen compounds for further study, from a group of fifty-nine candidate chemicals. Those twelve substances are caffeine; dietary supplements coenzyme Q10 (CoQ10) and creatine; estrogen (17-beta-estradiol), which is a hormone; GM-1 ganglioside; GPI-1485, minocycline, an antibiotic; nicotine; dopamine agonists pramipexole and ropinerole; and two drugs that are selective monoamine oxidase (MAO-B) inhibitors: rasagiline and selegiline.[1]

NEW USES FOR OLD DRUGS

Ibuprofen, the over-the-counter medication that so many of us take for headache and other minor pains, may also have neuroprotective qualities. Ibuprofen is in a class of drugs called "nonsteroidal anti-inflammatory drugs" (NSAIDs). In a study funded by the Michael J. Fox Foundation for Parkinson's Research and the NINDS, researchers found that people who took ibuprofen on a daily basis were 39 percent less likely to develop PD than those who took aspirin, another type of NSAIDs.[2]

Drugs to help you cope with PD

The following medications have made it through the FDA approval process in 2004 and are now available with a prescription from your physician. Depending upon where you live and the number of others with PD in your area, your pharmacy may have to place a special order, because the products are new.

Parcopa® is carbidopa/levodopa that dissolves in your mouth. It is especially useful if you have swallowing or choking problems or if you are a busy person who is frequently out and about without access to liquids (although you should always try to have a bottle of water with you to stay hydrated). Some people take Parcopa if they need levodopa during the night and don't want to drink water. Even if you don't take it on a regular basis, you might want to have a sample pack or two in your purse or glove compartment if you take Sinemet. You never know when you might need to take your medication when you are traveling or in a meeting or at church. It is also useful before surgical procedures when you can't drink water. (Take it from me—it is possible to take Sinemet by chewing it up without liquid. It doesn't have a bad taste, but it will not get into your system as quickly.)

Apomorphine (Apokyn®) is a drug designed to help individuals who have frequent freezing episodes or abrupt "off" times. This medication is administered by injection, and the dose needs to be titrated (calculated for your body weight and age). It also causes severe nausea, so an anti-emetic (a drug to prevent vomiting) is included in the injection.

Since "off" times usually occur after you've has been on Sinemet for several years, you probably won't be offered apomorphine for a while. However, you should know that it could be an option for you if you reach that point years from now.

Therapies in the future

RASAGILINE

Rasagiline is an MAO-B inhibitor that is currently being used in clinical trials. It is being tried alone (also known as **monotherapy**) and in conjunction with Sinemet. People with Parkinson's taking rasagiline showed much less progression of the PD than those taking a placebo.[3]

CELL THERAPY

A variety of different efforts that are under way involve the introduction of cells into the brain to produce dopamine or other brain chemicals that could alleviate symptoms of PD.

In theory, these ideas seem sound, but in practice, many have been surrounded by controversy and implementation problems. For example, hundreds of people with PD around the world have received transplants of fetal substantia nigra cells. Yet two showed that the only patient group that consistently showed improvement was that of the under-age-sixty participants, and many experienced significant side effects.[4] And any time human fetal cells are used, there are ethical issues and considerable public debate to contend with, because the cells are taken from aborted fetuses.

GLIAL CELL-DERIVED NEUROTROPHIC FACTOR (GDNF)

Another cell therapy, glial cell-derived neurotrophic factor (GDNF), has shown great promise in animal trials, but the results in people are mixed. GDNF is a protein that we produce in our central nervous system.[5] It is believed to protect dopaminergic neurons and possibly even to promote the growth of new ones, so you can understand why this could be a great tool against PD!

Yet, in October 2004, a biotechnology firm called Amgen, which had conducted several research trials of GDNF, announced that it was discontinuing the trials and that the compound would not be made available to study participants. The company said the compound had apparently damaged the brains of several monkeys that had received GDNF during research, and that some of the people with PD who had been given the drug had developed antibodies to it.[6] At this time, a number of study participants have filed a lawsuit against Amgen, requesting that they be allowed to continue to receive the therapy because they found it very beneficial. Information on the lawsuit, as well as testimonials from people with PD, can be found at www.gdnf4parkinsons.org/, a Web site put together by people with Parkinson's and families of many of the GDNF Phase I and Phase II research trial participants.

STEM CELL THERAPY

Stem cells are a bit like Legos for the body: they may not look like much, but you can make them into almost anything. These cells have not completely differentiated; that is, they haven't yet decided which type of cell they want to be when they grow up. Researchers are figuring out ways to influence that decision and get stem cells to become the types of cells needed to repair or cure many major diseases or conditions.

There are two categories of stem cells: embryonic and adult. Both types have shown promising results for treating Parkinson's disease or other health problems. Both types also have significant drawbacks that will need to be overcome if therapies are going to be realized anytime soon.

Embryonic Stem Cells

These cells can become any type of cell. Embryonic stem cells for research are currently obtained using embryos scheduled to be discarded by in vitro fertilization (IVF) clinics and have the full informed consent of the embryo donors.[7] There are at least two major physical disadvantages of embryonic stem cells. One is that if the embryo does not come from the patient receiving the cells, there is a chance that the cells will be rejected. The other is that because embryonic stem cells can become any type of cell, there are cases of tumors—clumps of undifferentiated cells called *teratomas*—being produced in lab animals receiving embryonic stem cells.[8]

Adult Stem Cells

Adult stem cells refer to any stem cells obtained after birth. This includes stem cells contained in the umbilical cord that connects a fetus to his or her mother. It is often called "cord blood." These cells are able to become more than one kind of cell within a certain type—e.g., blood cells, nerve cells, etc.[9] This makes them less versatile than embryonic stem cells. However, these cells can be taken from live donors and sometimes even the person who needs the cells. Bone marrow transplants are examples of adult stem cell transplants that have been going on for a long time.

The stem cell issues are very complex and ever changing. To learn more about the implications for stem cells and PD, I have listed in Resources a number of organizations relating to such research.

These issues bring with them moral and ethical questions that each of us must research and decide for ourself. I really do urge you to learn more about these promising therapies and then support the ones that you can, if any, by contacting your legislators.

IN A SENTENCE:

> *Pharmaceutical manufacturers, biotechnology companies, and medical device manufacturers are developing new treatments to prevent PD or alleviate the symptoms of Parkinson's disease.*

Appendix 1
Drug Diary and Drug Chart

Drug Diary

Commercial name of medication:	Generic name:
Prescribing physician:	Illness or condition being treated:
Symptoms drug is intended to treat:	Dosage: (example: 100 milligrams twice daily)
Duration of prescription (how long will you be taking it?)	Special dosing instructions:

Listed potential side effects (from medicine bottle or product info):		

Date taken:	Feelings/symptoms experienced today:	Other changes I noticed today:

Drug Chart

Drug	Common/ commercial name	Type	Stage of disease at which it is used	Symptoms it treats
Amantadine	Symmetrel	anti-viral	early use helps to reduce "on-off" periods; used in intermediate and later stages to help reduce dyskinesia	dyskinesia caused by Sinemet; poor balance
Apomorphine	Apokyn		intermediate-late	injectable drug that provides "instant on"—for use only with freezing epi-sodes or extreme "off" times
benztropine	cogentin	anti-cholinergic	had been pre-scribed before Sinemet was devel-oped; now not used much	suppresses ace-tylcholine (dopa-mine's "dance partner") to keep that neurotransmit-ter from becoming even more out-of-balance with the dopamine system
Bromocriptine	Parlodel	dopamine agonist	all	tremors; makes effects of Sinemet last longer and ease "on-off"periods
Cabergoline		ergoline dopa-mine agonist	early as monother-apy (taken alone); intermediate with levodopa	reduces "off" time, improves motor function, decreases need for levodopa

Symptoms it does NOT treat	Side effects	Known interactions with other drugs, foods, or other factors	Special instructions
	edema; skin problems; blurred vision; depression		
	dyskinesia; hallucinations; orthostatic hypotension ["Apomorphine: North American clinical experience." Mark Stacy, MD. NEUROLOGY 2004;62:S-18-S21		Must take anti-emetic (to prevent vomiting) or you WILL throw up
tremor; rigidity	dry mouth; constipation; rigidity; confusion; hallucinations; memory loss; blurred vision		
rigidity; slowness of movement	drowsiness, sometimes without warning; dizziness; nausea, vomiting; paranoia; hallucinations; confusion; dyskinesia; nightmares		For some patients, eating foods high in protein (e.g., meat, poultry, fish, dairy products, nuts) interferes with Sinemet absorption. If this happens, your health-care provider may recommend that you have most of your daily protein intake at your evening meal.
			Longest-acting DA, can be taken once/day

Drug	Common/ commercial name	Type	Stage of disease at which it is used	Symptoms it treats
carbidopa-levodopa	Atamet (generic)	dopamine precursor		rigidity; brady-kinesia (slowness of movement); gait (walking); facial masking; micrographica (small, cramped handwriting)
Carbidopa-Levodopa (oral dissolving)	Parcopa	dopamine precursor	intermediate-late	rigidity; brady-kinesia (slowness of movement); gait (walking); facial masking; micro-graphica (small, cramped hand-writing)
entacapone	Comtan	catechol-O-methyltransferase (COMT) inhibitor	early, late	suppresses COMT, which allows more levodopa to cross the blood-brain barrier
carbidopa-Levodopa	Sinemet; Atamet (generic version of Sinemet)	dopamine replacement	early (sometimes); intermediate; late	rigidity; brady-kinesia (slowness of movement)
Pergolide	Permax	dopamine agonist	all	tremors; makes effects of Sinemet last longer and ease "on-off" periods

Symptoms it does NOT treat	Side effects	Known interactions with other drugs, foods, or other factors	Special instructions
tremor; poor balance; speech problems; sexual dysfunction; pain; numbness & tingling; skin problems; gastrointestinal problems; depression/anxiety; dementia	nausea; vomiting; cardiac arrhythmia (irregular heartbeat); orthostatic hypotension (low blood pressure); dizziness; restlessness; dyskinesias (uncontrolled involuntary movements such as nodding, jerking, twitching); freezing; hallucinations; sleepiness		
tremor; poor balance; speech problems; sexual dysfunction; pain; numbness & tingling; skin problems; gastrointestinal problems; depression/anxiety; dementia	same potential side effects as Sinemet	This drug just became widely available in 2004.	useful for patients who have difficulty with swallowing/choking; also helpful for travel or people still working, because it can be taken without water
motor fluctuations			
tremors; poor balance	nausea; vomiting; cardiac arrhythmia (irregular heartbeat); orthostatic hypotension (low blood pressure); dizziness; restlessness; mental changes; Dyskinesias (uncontrolled involuntary movements such as nodding, jerking, twitching); freezing	Protein may interfere with absorption of the drug, especially after the patient has been on it for a long period of time.	"wearing off"—Medication's effects subside and symptoms resume. Physicians and patients strive to find a medication schedule that times doses frequently enough to avoid "off" times but not so much medication or so frequently that dyskinesias occur. The longer one is on Sinemet, the harder this balance is to achieve.
rigidity; slowness of movement	drowsiness, sometimes without warning; dizziness; nausea, vomiting; paranoia; hallucinations; confusion; dyskinesia; nightmares		sometimes used to treat "restless legs syndrome" (RLS)

Drug	Common/commercial name	Type	Stage of disease at which it is used	Symptoms it treats
Pramixerole	Mirapex	dopamine agonist	all	tremors; makes effects of Sinemet last longer and ease "on-off"periods
Ropinerole	Requip	dopamine agonist	all	tremors; makes effects of Sinemet last longer and ease "on-off" periods
Selegiline	Eldepryl	MAO inhibitor (prevents mono-amine oxidase B (MAO-B), a naturally occur-ring enzyme, from doing its job of breaking down dopamine	early	used to delay need for Sinemet (A study by the National Institutes for Neurologi-cal Diseases and Stroke (NINDS) found that sele-giline can post-pone the need for Sinemet by an average of nine months.); prolongs efficacy of Sinemet, eases "on-off" periods
trihexyphenidyl	Artane	anti-cholinergic	had been prescribed before Sinemet was devel-oped; now not used much	suppresses ace-tylcholine (dopa-mine's "dance partner") to keep that neurotransmit-ter from becoming even more out-of-balance with the dopamine system; sometimes taken with Sinemet or bromocriptine
carbidopa, entacapone & levodopa	Stalevo	dopamine replacement + anti-dyskinesia		
	provigil			
	resperidol			

Symptoms it does NOT treat	Side effects	Known interactions with other drugs, foods, or other factors	Special instructions
rigidity; slowness of movement	drowsiness, sometimes without warning; dizziness; nausea, vomiting; paranoia; hallucinations; confusion; dyskinesia; nightmares		sometimes used to treat "restless legs syndrome" (RLS)
rigidity; slowness of movement	drowsiness, sometimes without warning; dizziness; nausea, vomiting; paranoia; hallucinations; confusion; dyskinesia; nightmares		sometimes used to treat "restless legs syndrome" (RLS)
	nausea; low blood pressure; insomnia (if taken late in the day)	Toxic reactions have occurred in some patients taking fluoxetine (Prozac) and meperidine (Demerol).	
tremor; rigidity	dry mouth; constipation; rigidity; confusion; hallucinations; memory loss; blurred vision	Artane seems to be helpful to only about half of PD patients. Confusion, hallucinations and memory problems more common in elderly patients. [Leader, p. 18].	
	nausea, vomiting, or decreased appetite;		
			constipation, dry mouth, or blurred vision
			hand tremor

Drug	Common/ commercial name	Type	Stage of disease at which it is used	Symptoms it treats
carbidopa, entacapone & levodopa *(continued)*	Paxil	selective serotonin-reuptake inhibi-tors (SSRI)		
	Prozac			
	Celexa			
	Lexapro			
	Wellbutrin			
	Zoloft			
levodopa	Larodopa	dopamine replacement		
carbidopa-levodopa (controlled release)	Sinemet CR	dopamine replacement		

Symptoms it does NOT treat	Side effects	Known interactions with other drugs, foods, or other factors	Special instructions
			muscle twitches
			dizziness or drowsiness
			insomnia, confusion, or nightmares
			agitation or anxiety
			darkening of urine, sweat, or saliva (may cause discoloration of clothing); or fatigue.
			Do not crush or chew!

Appendix 2

Unified Parkinson's Disease Rating Scale

I. MENTATION, BEHAVIOR, AND MOOD

1. Intellectual Impairment
   0 = None.
   1 = Mild. Consistent forgetfulness with partial recollection of events and no other difficulties.
   2 = Moderate memory loss, with disorientation and moderate difficulty handling complex problems. Mild but definite impairment of function at home with need of occasional prompting.
   3 = Severe memory loss with disorientation for time and often to place. Severe impairment in handling problems.
   4 = Severe memory loss with orientation preserved to person only. Unable to make judgments or solve problems. Requires much help with personal care. Cannot be left alone at all.

2. Thought Disorder (due to dementia or drug intoxication)

0 = None.

1 = Vivid dreaming.

2 = "Benign" hallucinations with insight retained.

3 = Occasional to frequent hallucinations or delusions; without insight, could interfere with daily activities.

4 = Persistent hallucinations, delusions, or florrid psychosis. Not able to care for self.

3. Depression

1 = Periods of sadness or guilt greater than normal, never sustained for days or weeks.

2 = Sustained depression (1 week or more).

3 = Sustained depression with vegetative symptoms (insomnia, anorexia, weight loss, loss of interest).

4 = Sustained depression with vegetative symptoms and suicidal thoughts or intent.

4. Motivation/Initiative

0 = Normal.

1 = Less assertive than usual; more passive.

2 = Loss of initiative or disinterest in elective (nonroutine) activities.

3 = Loss of initiative or disinterest in day-to-day (routine) activities.

4 = Withdrawn, complete loss of motivation.

II. ACTIVITIES OF DAILY LIVING (FOR BOTH "ON" AND "OFF")

5. Speech

0 = Normal.

1 = Mildly affected. No difficulty being understood.

2 = Moderately affected. Sometimes asked to repeat statements.

3 = Severely affected. Frequently asked to repeat statements.

4 = Unintelligible most of the time.

6. Salivation

0 = Normal.

1 = Slight but definite excess of saliva in mouth; may have nighttime drooling.

2 = Moderately excessive saliva; may have minimal drooling.

3 = Marked excess of saliva with some drooling.

4 = Marked drooling, requires constant tissue or handkerchief.

7. Swallowing

0 = Normal.

1 = Rare choking.

2 = Occasional choking.

3 = Requires soft food.

4 = Requires NG tube or gastrotomy feeding.

8. Handwriting

0 = Normal.

1 = Slightly slow or small.

2 = Moderately slow or small; all words are legible.

3 = Severely affected; not all words are legible.

4 = The majority of words are not legible.

9. Cutting Food and Handling Utensils

0 = Normal.

1 = Somewhat slow and clumsy, but no help needed.

2 = Can cut most foods, although clumsy and slow; some help needed.

3 = Food must be cut by someone, but can still feed slowly.

4 = Needs to be fed.

10. Dressing

0 = Normal.

1 = Somewhat slow, but no help needed.

2 = Occasional assistance needed with buttoning, getting arms in sleeves.

3 = Considerable help required, but can do some things alone.

4 = Helpless.

11. Hygiene
0 = Normal.
1 = Somewhat slow, but no help needed.
2 = Needs help to shower or bathe; or very slow in hygienic care.
3 = Requires assistance for washing, brushing teeth, combing hair, going to bathroom.
4 = Foley catheter or other mechanical aids.

12. Turning in Bed and Adjusting Bed Clothes
0 = Normal.
1 = Somewhat slow and clumsy, but no help needed.
2 = Can turn alone or adjust sheets, but with great difficulty.
3 = Can initiate, but not turn or adjust sheets alone.
4 = Helpless.

13. Falling (unrelated to freezing)
0 = None.
1 = Rare falling.
2 = Occasionally falls, less than once per day.
3 = Falls an average of once daily.
4 = Falls more than once daily.

14. Freezing When Walking
0 = None.
1 = Rare freezing when walking; may have start hesitation.
2 = Occasional freezing when walking.
3 = Frequent freezing. Occasionally falls from freezing.
4 = Frequent falls from freezing.

15. Walking
0 = Normal.
1 = Mild difficulty. May not swing arms or may tend to drag leg.
2 = Moderate difficulty, but requires little or no assistance.
3 = Severe disturbance of walking, requiring assistance.
4 = Cannot walk at all, even with assistance.

16. **Tremor** (symptomatic complaint of tremor in any part of body.)
0 = Absent.
1 = Slight and infrequently present.
2 = Moderate; bothersome to patient.
3 = Severe; interferes with many activities.
4 = Marked; interferes with most activities.

17. **Sensory Complaints Related to Parkinsonism**
0 = None.
1 = Occasionally has numbness, tingling, or mild aching.
2 = Frequently has numbness, tingling, or aching; not distressing.
3 = Frequent painful sensations.
4 = Excruciating pain.

III. MOTOR EXAMINATION

18. **Speech**
0 = Normal.
1 = Slight loss of expression, diction or volume.
2 = Monotone, slurred but understandable; moderately impaired.
3 = Marked impairment, difficult to understand.
4 = Unintelligible.

19. **Facial Expression**
0 = Normal.
1 = Minimal hypomimia, could be normal "poker face".
2 = Slight but definitely abnormal diminution of facial expression
3 = Moderate hypomimia; lips parted some of the time.
4 = Masked or fixed facies with severe or complete loss of facial expression; lips parted ¼ inch or more.

20. Tremor at Rest (head, upper and lower extremities)

0 = Absent.

1 = Slight and infrequently present.

2 = Mild in amplitude and persistent. Or moderate in amplitude, but only intermittently present.

3 = Moderate in amplitude and present most of the time.

4 = Marked in amplitude and present most of the time.

21. Action or Postural Tremor of Hands

0 = Absent.

1 = Slight; present with action.

2 = Moderate in amplitude, present with action.

3 = Moderate in amplitude with posture holding as well as action.

4 = Marked in amplitude; interferes with feeding.

22. Rigidity (judged on passive movement of major joints with patient relaxed in sitting position; cogwheeling to be ignored)

0 = Absent.

1 = Slight or detectable only when activated by mirror or other movements.

2 = Mild to moderate.

3 = Marked, but full range of motion easily achieved.

4 = Severe, range of motion achieved with difficulty.

23. Finger Taps (patient taps thumb with index finger in rapid succession)

0 = Normal.

1 = Mild slowing or reduction in amplitude.

2 = Moderately impaired. Definite and early fatiguing. May have occasional arrests in movement.

3 = Severely impaired. Frequent hesitation in initiating movements or arrests in ongoing movement.

4 = Can barely perform the task.

24. Hand Movements (patient opens and closes hands in rapid succession)

0 = Normal.

1 = Mild slowing or reduction in amplitude.

2 = Moderately impaired. Definite and early fatiguing. May have occasional arrests in movement.

3 = Severely impaired. Frequent hesitation in initiating movements or arrests in ongoing movement.

4 = Can barely perform the task.

25. Rapid Alternating Movements of Hands (pronation-supination movements of hands, vertically and horizontally, with as large an amplitude as possible, both hands simultaneously)

0 = Normal.

1 = Mild slowing or reduction in amplitude.

2 = Moderately impaired. Definite and early fatiguing. May have occasional arrests in movement.

3 = Severely impaired. Frequent hesitation in initiating movements or arrests in ongoing movement.

4 = Can barely perform the task.

26. Leg Agility (patient taps heel on the ground in rapid succession picking up entire leg; amplitude should be at least 3 inches)

0 = Normal.

1 = Mild slowing or reduction in amplitude.

2 = Moderately impaired. Definite and early fatiguing. May have occasional arrests in movement.

3 = Severely impaired. Frequent hesitation in initiating movements or arrests in ongoing movement.

4 = Can barely perform the task.

27. **Arising from Chair** (patient attempts to rise from a straight-backed chair, with arms folded across chest)

0 = Normal.

1 = Slow; or may need more than one attempt.

2 = Pushes self up from arms of seat.

3 = Tends to fall back and may have to try more than one time, but can get up without help.

4 = Unable to arise without help.

28. **Posture**

0 = Normal erect.

1 = Not quite erect, slightly stooped posture; could be normal for older person.

2 = Moderately stooped posture, definitely abnormal; can be slightly leaning to one side.

3 = Severely stooped posture with kyphosis; can be moderately leaning to one side.

4 = Marked flexion with extreme abnormality of posture.

29. **Gait**

0 = Normal.

1 = Walks slowly, may shuffle with short steps, but no festination (hastening steps) or propulsion.

2 = Walks with difficulty, but requires little or no assistance; may have some festination, short steps, or propulsion.

3 = Severe disturbance of gait, requiring assistance.

4 = Cannot walk at all, even with assistance.

30. **Postural Stability** (response to sudden, strong posterior displacement produced by pull on shoulders while patient is erect with eyes open and feet slightly apart; patient is prepared.)

0 = Normal.

1 = Retropulsion, but recovers unaided.

2 = Absence of postural response; would fall if not caught by examiner.

3 = Very unstable, tends to lose balance spontaneously.

4 = Unable to stand without assistance.

31. **Body Bradykinesia and Hypokinesia** (combining slowness, hesitancy, decreased arm-swing, small amplitude, and poverty of movement in general)

0 = None.

1 = Minimal slowness, giving movement a deliberate character; could be normal for some persons. Possibly reduced amplitude.

2 = Mild degree of slowness and poverty of movement that is definitely abnormal. Alternatively, some reduced amplitude.

3 = Moderate slowness, poverty or small amplitude of movement.

4 = Marked slowness, poverty or small amplitude of movement.

IV. Complications of Therapy (In the past week)

A. *Dyskinesias*

32. **Duration: What proportion of the waking day are dyskinesias present?** (historical information)

0 = None.

1 = 1–25% of day.

2 = 26–50% of day.

3 = 51–75% of day.

4 = 76–100% of day.

33. **Disability: How disabling are the dyskinesias?** (historical information; may be modified by office examination)

0 = Not disabling.

1 = Mildly disabling.

2 = Moderately disabling.

3 = Severely disabling.

4 = Completely disabled.

34. **Painful Dyskinesias: How painful are the dyskinesias?**

0 = No painful dyskinesias.

1 = Slight.

2 = Moderate.

3 = Severe.

4 = Marked.

35. Presence of Early Morning Dystonia (historical information)

    0 = No

    1 = Yes

B. Clinical Fluctuations

36. Are "off" periods predictable?

    0 = No

    1 = Yes

37. Are "off" periods unpredictable?

    0 = No

    1 = Yes

38. Do "off" periods come on suddenly, within a few seconds?

    0 = No

    1 = Yes

39. What proportion of the waking day is the patient "off" on average?

    0 = None.

    1 = 1–25% of day.

    2 = 26–50% of day.

    3 = 51–75% of day.

    4 = 76–100% of day.

C. Other Complications

40. Does the patient have anorexia, nausea, or vomiting?

    0 = No

    1 = Yes

41. Any sleep disturbances, such as insomnia or hypersomnolence?

    0 = No

    1 = Yes

42. Does the patient have symptomatic orthostasis? (record the patient's blood pressure, height, and weight on the scoring form)

0 = No

1 = Yes

V. MODIFIED HOEHN AND YAHR STAGING

STAGE 0 =   No signs of disease.

STAGE 1 =   Unilateral disease.

STAGE 1.5 =   Unilateral plus axial involvement.

STAGE 2 =   Bilateral disease, without impairment of balance.

STAGE 2.5 =   Mild bilateral disease, with recovery on pull test.

STAGE 3 =   Mild to moderate bilateral disease; some postural instability; physically independent.

STAGE 4 =   Severe disability; still able to walk or stand unassisted.

STAGE 5 =   Wheelchair bound or bedridden unless aided.

VI. SCHWAB AND ENGLAND ACTIVITIES OF DAILY LIVING SCALE

100% = Completely independent. Able to do all chores without slowness, difficulty, or impairment. Essentially normal. Unaware of any difficulty.

90% = Completely independent. Able to do all chores with some degree of slowness, difficulty, and impairment. Might take twice as long. Beginning to be aware of difficulty.

80% = Completely independent in most chores. Takes twice as long. Conscious of difficulty and slowness.

70% = Not completely independent. More difficulty with some chores. Three to four times as long in some. Must spend a large part of the day with chores.

60% = Some dependency. Can do most chores, but exceedingly slowly and with much effort. Errors; some impossible.

50% = More dependent. Help with half, slower, etc. Difficulty with everything.

40% = Very dependent. Can assist with all chores, but few alone.

30% = With effort, now and then does a few chores alone or begins alone. Much help needed.

20% = Nothing alone. Can be a slight help with some chores. Severe invalid.

10% = Totally dependent, helpless. Complete invalid.

0% = Vegetative functions such as swallowing, bladder and bowel functions are not functioning. Bedridden.

Unified Parkinsons Disease Data Form

Name:

Unit Number:

Date:

DOPA mg/day		On	Off	On	Off	On	Off	On	Off	On	Off	On	Off	On	Off	On	Off
hrs DOPA lasts																	
1	Mentation																
2	Thought Disorder																
3	Depression																
4	Motivation/Initiative																
Subtotal: 1–4 (maximum=16)																	
5	Speech																
6	Salivation																
7	Swallowing																
8	Handwriting																
9	Cutting food																
10	Dressing																
11	Hygiene																
12	Turning in bed																
13	Falling																
14	Freezing																
15	Walking																
16	Tremor																
17	Sensory symptoms																
Subtotal: 5–17 (maximum=52)																	

Date:

	On	Off	On	Off	On	Off	On	Off	On	Off	On	Off	On	Off	On	Off
18 Speech																
19 Facial expression																
20 Tremor at rest: face, lips, chin																
Hands: right																
left																
Feet: right																
left																
21 Action tremor: right																
left																
22 Rigidity: neck																
Upper extremity: right																
left																
Lower extremity: right																
left																
23 Finger taps: right																
left																
24 Hand grips: right																
left																
25 Hand pronate/supinate: right																
left																
26 Leg agility: right																
left																
27 Arise from chair																
28 Posture																
29 Gait																
30 Postural stability																

Date:

	On	Off	On	Off	On	Off	On	Off	On	Off	On	Off	On	Off	On	Off
31 Body bradykinesia																
Subtotal: 18–31 (maximum=108)																
Total points: 1–31 (max=176)																
32 Dyskinesia (duration)																
33 Dyskinesia (disability)																
34 Dyskinesia (pain)																
35 Early morning dystonia																
36 "Offs" (predictable)																
37 "Offs" (unpredictable)																
38 "Offs" (sudden)																
39 "Offs" (duration)																
40 Anorexia, nausea, vomiting																
41 Sleep disturbance																
42 Symptomatic orthostasis																
Blood Pressure: seated																
supine																
standing																
Weight																
Pulse: seated																
standing																

Name of examiner:

	Best	Worst	Best	Worst	Best	Worst	Best	Worst	Best	Worst	Best	Worst	Best	Worst	Best	Worst
Hoehn & Yahr Stage																
% ADL Score (PD)																
% ADL (with dyskinesia)																

Fahn S, Elton R, Members of the UPDRS Development Committee. In: Fahn S, Marsden CD, Calne DB, Goldstein M, eds. Recent Developments in Parkinson's Disease, Vol 2. Florham Park NJ. Macmillan Health Care Information 1987, pp. 153–163, 293–304

Appendix 3

THE PD SURVEY

WHEN I was asked to write this book, it had already been a few years since I had been newly diagnosed. I didn't want to rely solely on my own recollections of what that experience was like. I also knew that many other people with Parkinson's disease and their care partners would have good advice and anecdotes to share.

I used Survey Monkey, an Internet survey tool (www.survey-monkey.com), to collect survey responses from December 8 through 31, 2004. I e-mailed a direct link to numerous friends with PD and urged them to circulate word about the survey, too. I received 151 responses, which was very surprising and exciting, given the short time frame.

This survey was not created using statistically valid techniques, nor was it intended to be used for research purposes. The following is an excerpted list of the survey questions, along with some response data. You should be aware that not all respondents answered all of the questions. I am including the response data because you may find it interesting, and so that you have demographic information about the survey respondents mentioned in this book.

What I wish I had known about Parkinson's disease

WHO IS DOING THIS SURVEY, AND WHY?

Hi. My Name is Jackie Christensen, I'm a 40-year-old wife, mom of two boys (13 and 8) and activist on health and environmental issues. I have had Parkinson's disease for at least 8 years.

Recently, I was asked to write a book on dealing with the first year of Parkinson's disease (PD).

I have been reflecting a lot about what I WISH that I had known when I was diagnosed or soon after. Rather than having the book mention only my experiences, I thought I should ask other people with Parkinson's disease— PWP for short—to add the information. I believe that this will make the book more useful and more interesting.

NOTE: By completing the survey, you are agreeing to allow me to use your answers to these survey questions in my book. If you choose to share an anecdote or experience with me, I will use either your first name only, or if you prefer, your initials.

I will NOT be collecting contact information except from those people willing to submit to a phone interview or those who would like to receive a postcard/notice when the book is available.

Please feel free to forward this survey to others impacted by Parkinson's disease. The only restrictions I am putting on the survey are that

- I will accept no more than 1000 responses
- all responses need to be in by December 31, 2004.

Thanks for your help in getting the word out!

ABOUT YOU: These questions will let me know some general things about your experiences with Parkinson's disease (PD). If you are not the person with PD, please think of that person's situation when answering this section.

1. Which selection describes your role in completing this survey?

	% response
I am a person with Parkinson's disease (PWP)	78.0%
I am a care partner (spouse or life partner)	12.4%
I am a care partner (non-family member)	0.7%
I am a child or close relative or friend of someone with PD but not the primary care partner	5.5%
I am a paid personal care attendant/home health aide	0%
I am a health care provider	5.5%
Other (please specify)	0.7%

2. How long have you (or the person with Parkinson's that you care for) had Parkinson's disease?

less than one year	5.4%
1–3 years	23%
3–5 years	16.2%
5–8 years	18.2%
more than 8 years	33.1%
not sure	4.1%

3. What was the approximate length of time between when you first consulted a health care provider about symptoms and when you received a diagnosis of Parkinson's disease?

**If you are not someone with PD, please skip ahead to question 13. Thanks.

At same appointment	20.7%
Within 3 months of my first visit	22.9%
3–6 months	13.6%
6–12 months	12.7%
1 year +	20.7%
not sure	10.7%

4. How old were you when you were diagnosed?

5. What type of health care practitioner made the PD diagnosis?

My primary care physician/family doctor	11.2%
A neurologist	81.3%
A movement disorder specialist	15.7%
Other (please specify)	6.7%

6. Do you feel that your health care provider gave you enough information about Parkinson's disease when she/he made the diagnosis?

Yes	38.6%
No	48.5%
Not sure	12.9%

7. Are you still being treated by the health care practitioner who made the diagnosis?

| Yes | 35.6% |
| No | 64.4% |

8. Are you taking any medication for your Parkinson's disease (including anti-depressants prescribed since you were diagnosed)?

| Yes | 92.6% |
| No | 7.4% |

9. Do you have any family history of Parkinson's disease or other movement disorders?

Yes	31%
No	56.3%
Not sure	12.7%

10. What type of medications are you taking? (check all that apply)

dopamine agonist (such as Mirapex, Permax, Requip)	68.9%
carbidopa/levodopa (Sinemet)	77.3%
anti-dyskinesia (such as Amantadine, Comtan)	29.5%
anti-depressant (such as Celexa, Lexapro, Paxil, Prozac, Wellbutrin, Zoloft)	38.6%
Other (please specify)	34.8%

11. How has Parkinson's disease affected your life so far?

	Response	% response
I have had to modify some of my favorite hobbies or activities.	Yes	83%
	No	15%
	Not applicable (N/A)	2%
I have had to stop some of my favorite hobbies or activities.	Yes	67%
	No	32%
	N/A	1%
I need help dressing myself.	Yes	23%
	No	77%
	N/A	0%
I have had to ask for accommodations or make changes in my job.	Yes	37%
	No	33%
	N/A	30%
I have had to stop working.	Yes	43%
	No	37%
	N/A	20%
I receive disability/supplemental Social Security payments.	Yes	29%
	No	66%
	N/A	5%

		Response	% response
I use assistive devices (such as a cane, a walker, tub transfer bench, specialized household items).		Yes	35%
		No	63%
		N/A	2%
I have trouble sleeping.		Yes	72%
		No	28%
		N/A	0%
I have trouble concentrating, focusing on tasks and/or remembering things like I used to.		Yes	69%
		No	31%
		N/A	0%
I have had to stop driving.		Yes	18%
		No	81%
		N/A	1%
I have had to move to a more accessible house/apartment.		Yes	13%
		No	85%
		N/A	2%
I have had to move to an assisted-living facility.		Yes	3%
		No	97%
		N/A	0%
I have had problems with my speech and/or had choking problems.		Yes	53%
		No	46%
		N/A	1%

12. Have you had, or are you considering, any brain-related surgery for PD (such as pallidotomy, thalamatomy, deep-brain stimulation)?

Yes, have had surgery (list type under "Other")	13%
Yes, am considering surgery (list type under "Other")	9.6%
No	77.4%
Other	22.6%

FOR PEOPLE WITH PARKINSON'S AS WELL AS CARE PARTNERS OR FAMILY MEMBERS/FRIENDS:

13. Do you attend a support group for people with PD and/or for care partners or children?

Yes	63.8%
No	27.5%
I would if there was one in my area.	8.7%

14. Have you contacted any of the national organizations that provide information and resources on PD?

Yes	94%
No	4%
Not sure	2%

If so, which ones have you contacted? Check all that apply

American Parkinson's Disease Association	57.9%
Michael J. Fox Foundation	51.9%
National Parkinson Foundation	77.6%
Parkinson's Action Network	30.4%
Parkinson's Alliance	15.9%
Parkinson's Disease Foundation	30.8%
Parkinson's Institute	9.8%
WE MOVE	16.8%
Other (Please specify)	21.5%

15. What were the most useful pieces of advice or information that you received within the first year of diagnosis?

16. Are there any facts or experiences that you know about now that you WISH someone would have told you during your first year with PD? Please list and give as many details as you are comfortable sharing.

17. Are there any facts or experiences that you learned when you were first diagnosed that you wish you HAD NOT learned? Please list and give as many details as you are comfortable sharing.

18. Are you willing to be contacted for a phone interview? (PLEASE NOTE THAT I MAY NOT BE ABLE TO CONTACT EVERYONE WHO VOLUNTEERS. I WILL CONTACT AS MANY PEOPLE AS POSSIBLE. THE MORE INFO YOU CAN GIVE IN OTHER QUESTIONS, THE MORE LIKELY I AM TO CONTACT YOU.)

19. Do you have any comments that you would like to make about the survey, or about your experiences with PD? If so, please add them here.

20. If you are willing to be contacted, please provide your first name (last name, if you wish), phone number with area code, and the best times and days to contact you.

    Name:

    Phone:

    Best time of day to contact me:

    Best day(s) of week to contact me:

21. How did you learn about the survey?

You e-mailed the link to me	28%
Someone forwarded the survey link to me	55.5%
Referral/Link from another site	5.5%
Other (please specify):	11%

22. Where do you live?

United States	99%
Other country	1%

23. If you are in the United States, please list your state.

Notes

Day 1

1. Nausieda and Bock, *Parkinson's Disease: What You and Your Family Should Know*, 7.
2. Parkinson's Disease Foundation, *Frequently Asked Questions About Parkinson's Disease*.
3. Parkinson's Action Network, "What Is Parkinson's Disease."
4. Lieberman, *Shaking Up Parkinson's Disease*, 125.
5. Lai and Tsui, "Epidemiology of Parkinson's Disease."
6. Jahanshahi and Marsden, *Parkinson's Disease: A Self-Help Guide*, 8.
7. "Parkinson's Disease (Shaking Palsy)," *Merck Manual of Diagnosis and Therapy*.
8. "How Does an MRI Work?"
9. Leader and Leader, *Parkinson's Disease—The Way Forward!*
10. Michael J. Fox Foundation for Parkinson's Research, "Michael J. Fox Foundation for Parkinson's Research to Fund Research for Parkinson's Biomarker."
11. Michael J. Fox Foundation, "New Test May Detect Parkinson's Early, Aid Search for Drugs."
12. Sharma and Richman, *Parkinson's Disease and the Family*, 118–19.

Day 2

1. Schuster, "Pessimism, Anxiety Tied to Development of Parkinson's Disease."
2. Pfeiffer, "Parkinson's Disease and Nonmotor Dysfunction."

3. University of Pennsylvania, "Olfactory Function in Relatives of Patients with Parkinson's Disease."
4. National Institute of Neurological Diseases and Stroke, "Parkinson's Disease: Hope Through Research."
5. NINDS and NIH, "Parkinson's Disease: Challenges, Progress and Promise."

Day 3

1. National Institute of Neurological Diseases and Stroke, "Parkinson's Disease: Hope Through Research."
2. Di Minno and Aminoff, "Treatment Options."
3. Hubble and Bertou, *Parkinson's Disease: Medications.*
4. Cerner Multum, Inc., "Tasmar."
5. Cerner Multum, Inc., "Selegiline."
6. Di Minno and Aminoff, *Parkinson's Disease: Medications.*
7. Körner, et al., "Predictors of Sudden Onset of Sleep in Parkinson's Disease."
8. Cummings, "A Window on the Role of Dopamine in Addiction Disorders."
9. Ali and Morley, "Treatment of Parkinson's Disease (PD)."
10. Lieberman, "What You Should Know About Young-Onset Parkinson Disease.
11. Hubble and Bertou, *Parkinson's Disease: Medications,* 7.
12. Holden, "Fava Beans, Levodopa and Parkinson's Disease."
13. Lieberman, "Parkinson Disease, Parkinson-Like, Parkinson-Plus."
14. Worldwide Education and Awareness for Movement Disorders (WE MOVE), "Overview of Multiple System Atrophy."
15. Lieberman, "Parkinson Disease, Parkinson-Like."
16. WE MOVE, "Overview of Progressive Supranuclear Palsy."
17. Lieberman, "Parkinson Disease, Parkinson-Like."
18. Marjama-Lyons and Shomon, *What Your Doctor May Not Tell You About Parkinson's Disease,* 261.

Day 4

1. NINDS, "Parkinson's Disease: Hope Through Research."
2. Greenamyre and Hastings, "Parkinson's—Divergent Causes, Convergent Mechanisms."
3. National Institute on Aging, "Scientists Detect Probable Genetic Cause of Parkinson's Disease."
4. Poorkaj, et al., "Parkin Mutation Dosage and the Phenomenon of Anticipation: A Molecular Genetic Study of Familial Parkinsonism."
5. Langston, "Accelerating Research on Genes and Environment in Parkinson's Disease."
6. Lieberman, "Parkinson Disease, Parkinson-Like."
7. Mayo Clinic—Jacksonville, Florida, "Mayo Clinic Researchers and Former Colleagues Find Cause."
8. Langston, "Accelerating Research on Genes and Environment in Parkison's Disease."
9. Lieberman, "Parkinson Disease, Parkinson-Like."
10. Marjama-Lyons and Shomon, *What Your Doctor May Not Tell You,* 28.
11. Lieberman, *Shaking Up Parkinson's Disease.*

12. Liu, et al., "Parkinson's Disease and Exposure to Infectious Agents."
13. Lieberman, *Shaking Up Parkinson's Disease,* 117.
14. Langston, et al., "Chronic Parkinsonism in Humans Due to a Product of Meperidine-Analog Synthesis."
15. Myers, "Gene Expression and Environmental Exposures: New Opportunities for Disease."

Day 5

1. Lieberman, *Shaking Up Parkinson's Disease,* 60.
2. Chong, "Levodopa-Induced Dyskinesias," 206–09
3. Cram, *Understanding Parkinson's Disease: A Self-Help Guide,* 54.
4. Pfeiffer, "Parkinson's Disease and Nonmotor Disease Function."
5. Kaasinen, et al., "Personality Traits and Brain Dopaminergic Function in Parkinson's Disease."
6. Salloway, "Neuropsychiatric Aspects of Movement Disorders;"
7. Gschwandtner, et al., "Pathologic Gambling in Patients with Parkinson's Disease." Sharma and Richman, *Parkinson's Disease and the Family,* 118-19.

Day 6

1. Lieberman, *Shaking Up Parkinson's Disease,* 158.
2. National Institutes of Mental Health, "Depression and Parkinson's Disease."

Week 2

1. Sierpina and Frenkel, "Acupuncture: A Clinical Review."
2. Saito, "The Shiatsu Story."
3. Shiatsu Academy of Tokyo, "A Brief History of Shiatsu."
4. "Different Types of Massage Therapy."
5. "Tai Chi and Yohimbine Could Help Parkinson's."
6. Ives and Sosnoff, "Beyond the Mind-Body Exercise Hype."
7. Jankovic, "What is the role of CoQ10 in the treatment of Parkinson's disease (PD)?"
8. "ConsumerLab.com Finds Discrepancies in Strengths of CoQ10 Supplements."
9. Parkinson's Disease Society, "Jane Asher Announces Parkinson's Awareness Week."
10. Lieberman, *Shaking Up Your Doctor: Getting the Most from Your Visit.*

Week 4

1. Cannuscio, et al., "Reverberation of Family Illness: A Longitudinal Assessment."

Month 3

1. Lee Silverman Voice Treatment Web site, www.lsvt.org/main_site.htm/.

Month 4

1. "Dietary Reference Intakes—Vitamins."
2. Holden, "Parkinson's, B_6, B_{12} and Folate—What's the Connection".
3. Ibid.

Month 5

1. Leader and Leader, *Parkinson's Disease: The Way Forward!* 121.

Month 7

1. "The Exercise and Fitness Page of Georgia State University."

Month 8

1. U.S. Department of Justice, "Americans with Disabilities Act / Questions and Answers."

Month 9

1. Mayo Clinic staff, "Dementia: Not Always Alzheimer's."
2. Merino, et al., "Parkinson's Disease Dementia."
3. Pfeiffer; Sharma & Richman, "Parkinson's Disease Q&A" patient information booklet, Parkinson's Disease Foundation; Blair Ford, MD, FRCP (C), Pietro Mazzoni, M.D., Ph.D., Panida Piboolnurak, MD. December 15, 2004.
4. Mayo Clinic Staff, "Dementia: Not Always Alzheimer's."

Month 10

1. Marjama-Lyons and Shomon, *What Your Doctor May Not Tell You*, 124–25.
2. NINDS, *Parkinson's Disease: A Research-Planning Workshop.*
3. Marjama-Lyons and Shomon, 123–24.
4. Ibid., 128.
5. NINDS, *Parkinson's Disease: A Research-Planning Workshop.*
6. Di Minno and Aminoff, *"Treatment Options."*
7. Ibid.
8. Ibid.
9. Medtronic, "Questions and Answers about Activa Parkinson's Control Therapy."
10. Marsh and Berk, "Neuropsychiatric Aspects of Parkinson's Disease: Recent Advances."

Month 11

1. Hungelmann, "What Young-Onset Persons with Parkinson's Need to Know About Insurance."

Month 12

1. Chen, "Neuroprotection in Parkinson's Disease."
2. Moyer, "Ibuprofen May Protect Against Parkinson's Disease."
3. Waknine, "Early Rasagiline Therapy Shows Long-Term Benefits for Parkinson's."
4. WE MOVE, "Experimental Therapies."
5. Parkinson's Pipeline Project, "Amgen Halts GDNF Trial: What's All the Controversy About?"
6. Amgen, Inc., "Following Complete Review of Phase 2 Trial Data Amgen Confirms Decision to Halt GDNF Study."
7. Stem Cell Institute, "Stem Cell 101."
8. National Institutes of Health, "Chapter 3: The Human Embryonic Stem Cell and Human Embryonic Germ Cell," 17.
9. Stem Cell Institute, "Stem Cell 101."

Glossary

ACETYLCHOLINE: A chemical messenger released by cholinergic nerves. Normally in many parts of the body, including the brain, and necessary to normal body functioning. There appears to be a reciprocal seesaw relationship between acetylcholine and dopamine and their respective nerve cell systems.

ACTION TREMOR: Rhythmic, involuntary movement of a limb when movement is initiated, e.g., when writing or lifting a cup. Not usually seen in the earlier stages of Parkinson's.

ACTIVITIES OF DAILY LIVING (ADLs): Routine activities that a person does on a daily basis, e.g., bathing, eating, brushing teeth, grooming, and hand washing.

ADRENALINE (EPINEPHRINE): The neurotransmitter of the adrenal gland that is secreted in moments of crisis. It stimulates the heart to beat faster and work harder, increases the flow of blood to the muscles, causes an increased alertness of mind, and produces other changes to prepare the body to meet an emergency.

AGONIST: A chemical or drug that mimics neurotransmitter activity.

AKINESIA: Absence of body movements.

ALPHA-SYNUCLEIN: A protein that is believed to have a causative role in Parkinson's. All human brains contain about 2 percent alpha-synuclein, but in PD patients it often forms clumps called Lewy bodies. The exact purpose of alpha-synuclein and whether the protein itself is harmful remain unknown.

AMANTADINE (SYMMETREL): A drug developed to prevent influenza that has been found to control dyskinesia. It may also be prescribed as a monotherapy in early Parkinson's disease to treat bradykinesia, rigidity, and tremors.

AMYOTROPHIC LATERAL SCLEROSIS (ALS): Degenerative neurological disease marked by the destruction of motor neurons in the brain. Also known as Lou Gehrig's disease because the legendary baseball star died from the disease.

ANTICHOLINERGIC: Referring to a substance (medication) that reduces the action of acetylcholine.

ANTIDEPRESSANT: Drug that is used to treat depression.

ANTIOXIDANT: Chemical compound that prevents free radicals from stealing electrons from cells within the body, thereby preventing cell death.

ANTICHOLINERGIC DRUGS (ARTANE, COGENTIN): The group of drugs that decrease the action of acetylcholine. The specified drugs may help reduce rigidity, tremor, and drooling in Parkinson's.

APOMORPHINE: A derivative of morphine and a dopamine agonist. Currently available in injectable form for freezing episodes in severe Parkinson's.

AUTONOMIC NERVOUS SYSTEM: The branch of the nervous system that controls internal organs in the body, i.e., heart, lungs.

BASAL GANGLIA OR NUCLEI: Deeper structures in the brain, concerned with normal movement and walking. The caudate nucleus, putamen, and substantia nigra are basal ganglia affected in Parkinson's.

BILATERAL: Occurring on both sides of the body.

BIOMARKER: A physical trait that is used to detect the presence of a disease or condition, or to evaluate its progression.

BLEPHAROSPASM: Spasmodic blinking or involuntary closing of the eye lids; a type of dystonia.

BRADYKINESIA: Slowing down of a movement. Bradykinesia involves slowness of initiating and executing movements and fine motor movements and difficulty in performing repetitive movements. It is a major symptom of Parkinson's.

CARBIDOPA: The ingredient in Sinemet that prevents the breakdown of the levodopa in the body before it can reach the brain.

CENTRAL NERVOUS SYSTEM (CNS): Consists of the brain and spinal cord.

CEREBELLUM: Area of the brain that controls complex muscle movements, posture, and balance.

CHOLINE: A naturally occurring substance that is a precursor of acetylcholine.

CLINICAL TRIAL: A research study to gather information about a disease, determine the efficacy of potential treatments, or identify the cause of a health condition. These studies are done prior to government approval of drugs or medical devices.

COGWHEEL RIGIDITY: Stiffness in the muscles, with a jerky quality when arm and leg joints are repeatedly moved.

COMPUTERIZED AXIAL TOMOGRAPHY SCAN (CAT OR CT SCAN): An imaging test that uses radiation to help doctors detect bleeding or bone problems in the body.

COMT INHIBITOR: Drug that prevents catechol-O-methyl transferase (COMT), an enzyme, from breaking down levodopa in the brain.

CONSTIPATION: Diminished ability of intestinal muscles to move feces (stool), often resulting in very hard stool. A common problem in Parkinson's.

CORPUS STRIATUM: Area of brain controlling movement, balance, and walking. Connects to and receives impulses from substantia nigra.

DARDARIN: Gene suspected as the cause of some cases of inherited Parkinson's.

DEEP-BRAIN STIMULATION (DBS): System of electrodes with a power supply that uses electrical impulses to reduce or eliminate many symptoms of Parkinson's disease. It can be targeted to specific regions of the brain to address particular symptoms.

DEGENERATIVE: Caused by deterioration or breakdown.

DEPRENYL (ELDEPRYL, SELEGILINE): A drug that slows the breakdown of chemicals like dopamine by inhibiting the action of certain enzymes. It increases effects of dopamine in the brain.

DEPRESSION: Mental state marked by extreme sadness, lack of motivation, and inability to concentrate.

DJ-1: Gene suspected as the cause of some cases of inherited Parkinson's.

DOPAMINE: A chemical produced by the brain; it assists in the effective transmission of electrochemical messages from one nerve cell to the next. It is deficient in the basal ganglia and substantia nigra of a person with Parkinson's. It governs actions of movement, balance, and walking.

DOPAMINE AGONIST: Drugs that mimic the effects of dopamine and stimulate the dopamine receptors.

DOPAMINERGIC: Referring to a chemical, a drug, or a drug effect related to dopamine.

DRUG DIARY: Document used to track dosage and effects of medications over time.

DRUG HOLIDAY: A period of time that marks the withdrawal of a drug after long-term treatment.

DRUG-INDUCED PARKINSONISM: Parkinson's symptoms that have been caused by drugs used to treat other conditions.

DYSARTHRIA: Speech difficulties caused when the muscles associated with speech are affected.

DYSKINESIA: A condition marked by the abnormal movement of voluntary muscles. Dystonia, athetosis, and chorea are types of dyskinesia.

DYSPHAGIA: Difficulty in swallowing.

DYSTONIA: Involuntary spasms of muscle contraction that cause abnormal movements and postures. May appear as a side effect of long-term drug treatment in Parkinson's and may worsen in response to stress.

ENCEPHALITIS: Inflammation of the brain, usually caused by a virus infection.

ENCEPHALITIS LETHARGICA (SLEEPING SICKNESS): A specific kind of encephalitis that occurred in scattered epidemics throughout the world during the period 1916 to 1926; it usually caused sleepiness, double vision, trouble swallowing, and drooling. Many of those affected developed advanced parkinsonism, as depicted in the movie *Awakenings*.

ESSENTIAL TREMOR: A condition characterized by tremor of the hands, head, voice, and sometimes other parts of the body. Essential tremor often runs in families and is sometimes called familial tremor. It is sometimes mistaken for a symptom of Parkinson's. However, this is an action tremor and there is no rigidity or bradykinesia.

FESTINATION: Walking in rapid, short, shuffling steps.

FREE RADICAL: Atom that has at least one free electron and therefore is very unstable. Free radicals can cause cell damage and may play a role in the causation of Parkinson's.

FREEZING: Temporary, involuntary inability to move.

GASTROINTESTINAL TRACT: The part of the digestive system that includes the stomach and large and small intestines.

GLOBUS PALLIDUS: The inner part of the lenticular nucleus. The lenticular nucleus and the caudate nucleus form the striatum.

HALLUCINATION: Experiences (sights, sounds) that are not real but are perceived as real.

HEAVY METAL: Element that is toxic or harmful to humans and animals.

HEIMLICH MANEUVER: A form of first aid for people who are choking.

HOMOCYSTEINE: An amino acid that is used to build proteins. It may play a role in the formation of Lewy bodies, the clumps of protein in the brain that are a hallmark of Parkinson's disease.

HYPOKINESIA: Abnormally diminished motor activity.

IDIOPATHIC: "Of unknown cause." The usual form of Parkinson's is idiopathic Parkinson's.

INFLAMMATION: The body's physical reaction to injury or infection, characterized by pain, swelling, redness, and possibly loss of function.

L-3,4-DIHYDROXYPHENYLALANINE (LEVODOPA): The international generic name for the medicinal formulation of L-dopa that is converted to dopamine once it crosses the blood-brain barrier. It is contained in Sinemet, Madopar, Parcopa, and other prescription dopamine replacements.

LEVODOPA-INDUCED DYSKINESIAS: A side effect of medication that may occur with prolonged use. These abnormal, involuntary movements may be alleviated by reducing the amount of medication.

LEWY BODY: Clumps of the protein alpha-synuclein that clutter the brain. They are considered markers for Parkinson's.

LIVEDO RETICULARIS: A condition of the circulatory system that is marked by purplish or bluish mottling of the skin. It is seen usually below the knee and sometimes on the forearm in persons under treatment with the drug amantadine (Symmetrel).

MADOPAR: Commercial name for levodopa medication marketed in Europe.

MANEB: A chemical mixture that combines manganese and a pesticide to kill fungus on fruits and vegetables. Exposure is linked to the development of Parkinson's disease later in life

MASKED FACE: Effect of rigidity in facial muscles that causes a blank, unemotional expression (like a mask).

1-METHYL-4-PHENYL-1,2,3,6-TETRAHYDROPYRIDINE (MPTP): A toxic chemical made by IV drug users attempting to synthesize heroin. It can induce PD-like symptoms in lab animals and is used in lab studies to test the PD-causing potential of different compounds.

MICROGRAPHIA: The tendency to have very small handwriting due to difficulty with fine motor movements in Parkinson's.

MITOCHONDRIA: Part of a cell that is responsible for generating the energy needed for healthy cell functioning.

MONOAMINE OXIDASE: Enzyme that breaks down dopamine, as well as other neurotransmitters (e.g., serotonin and epinephrine.)

MONOAMINE OXIDASE INHIBITOR: Drug that blocks the action of monoamine enzymes, thus allowing dopamine to circulate in the brain longer.

MONOTHERAPY: When a drug is used alone for treatment of a condition or disease, instead of in combination with other medications.

MOTOR CORTEX: Part of the brain in which nerve impulses that control muscle movements originate.

MULTIPLE SCLEROSIS: A disease that occurs when lesions are formed on the outer covering of the nerve fibers in the brain and the spinal column. It has many symptoms in common with Parkinson's disease.

MYOCLONUS: Jerking, involuntary movement of arms and legs, usually occurring during sleep.

NATIONAL CENTER FOR COMPLEMENTARY AND ALTERNATIVE MEDICINE (NCCAM): Division of the NIH that funds and oversees research into complementary therapies.

NATIONAL INSTITUTES OF HEALTH (NIH): Federal agency that allocates funding for human health-related research in the United States and supervises that research.

NEURON: A cell in the nervous system that conducts impulses to the brain, spinal column, or nerves.

NEUROTRANSMITTER: A specialized chemical produced in nerve cells that permits the transmission of information between nerve cells.

NOREPINEPHRINE (NORADRENALIN): Chemical transmitter found mainly in two areas of the brain involved in governing the involuntary autonomic nervous system.

NORMAL PRESSURE HYDROCEPHALUS: A condition marked by an increase in the amount of spinal fluid in the brain. It can cause neurological symptoms similar to Parkinson's.

"OFF" TIME: Slang phrase used to refer to periods when Parkinson's medications are not alleviating symptoms of rigidity, tremor, slowed movements, or poor balance.

OLIVOPONTOCEREBELLAR ATROPHY: A form of parkinsonism marked by significant changes in balance and coordination. Considered to be a "Parkinson's Plus" disorder.

ON-OFF FLUCTUATIONS: Fluctuations that occur in response to levodopa therapy in which the person's mobility changes suddenly and unpredictably from a good response (on) to a poor response (off).

ORTHOSTATIC HYPOTENSION: A drop in blood pressure during rapid changes in body position (e.g., from sitting to standing). Many medications for Parkinson's may cause or exacerbate this condition.

OVER-THE-COUNTER MEDICINE (OTCs): Drugs that are available for purchase without a prescription.

OXIDATION: Process in which the presence of oxygen allows free radicals to steal electrons—a situation that causes chemical reactions that can lead to cell death.

PALLIDOTOMY: Irreversible surgery in which a lesion is formed to destroy part of the globus pallidus to alleviate PD symptoms.

PARAESTHESIA: Sensations, usually unpleasant, arising spontaneously in a limb or other part of the body, variously experienced as a prickly feeling (pins and needles) or a feeling of warmth or coldness (thermal paresthesias).

PARASYMPATHETIC NERVOUS SYSTEM: The part of the autonomic nervous system originating in the brain stem and the lower part of the spinal cord that, in general, inhibits or opposes the physiological effects of the sympathetic nervous system, as in tending to stimulate digestive secretions or slow the heart.

PARKIE: Slang or familiar term for person with Parkinson's disease.

PARKIN: Gene suspected in some cases of Parkinson's disease that may be due to heredity.

PARKINSONIAN: Term that refers to someone with Parkinson's disease or an adjective describing something related to Parkinson's disease or parkinsonism.

PARKINSON'S DISEASE: That form of parkinsonism originally described by James Parkinson as a chronic, slowly progressive disease of the nervous system characterized clinically by the combination of tremor, rigidity, bradykinesia, and stooped posture, and pathologically by loss of the pigmented nerve cells of the substantia nigra in the brain.

PARKINSONISM: A clinical state characterized by tremor, rigidity, bradykinesia, stooped posture, and shuffling gait. The more common causes of parkinsonism are Parkinson's disease, striatonigral degeneration, and a reversible syndrome induced by major tranquilizing drugs.

PARKINSON'S PLUS (PD+) SYNDROMES: Forms of parkinsonism that may be initially diagnosed as Parkinson's disease. They generally do not respond to treatment with levodopa (Sinemet).

PARLODEL (BROMOCRIPTINE): A dopamine agonist useful in treating all of the primary symptoms of Parkinson's. It may be used alone or with other antiparkinson medications.

PERMAX (PERGOLIDE): A dopamine agonist similar in action to Parlodel but more potent.

PESTICIDE: A substance used to kill undesirable living things (e.g., plants, insects, fungi and rodents).

PLACEBO: A substitute compound that does not contain an active ingredient or medication but is intended to convince the patient that it is real, to raise their expectations of getting well.

POSITRON EMISSION TOMOGRAPHY SCAN (PET SCAN): An imaging technology that can be used to diagnose Parkinson's Plus syndromes, such as multiple system atrophy and progressive supranuclear palsy. It was invented in 1981.

POSTURAL DEFORMITY: Stooped posture.

POSTURAL INSTABILITY: Difficulty with balance.

POSTURAL TREMOR: Tremor that increases when hands are stretched out in front.

PRECURSOR: Something that precedes, e.g., a sign or symptom that forewarns of another, such as muscle aching may be the precursor of a tremor. Can also refer to a substance that is an ingredient in a more stable mixture.

PROGRESSIVE SUPRANUCLEAR PALSY (PSP): A degenerative brain disorder sometimes difficult to distinguish from Parkinson's, especially in the early stages. PSP symptoms are rigidity and akinesia, difficulty looking up and down, and speech and balance problems. Those with PSP often have poor response to antiparkinson medications.

PROPULSIVE GAIT: Disturbance of gait typical of parkinsonism in which, during walking, steps become faster and faster with progressively shorter steps that pass from a walking to a running pace and may precipitate falling forward.

RANGE OF MOTION: The extent that a joint will move from being fully straightened to completely bent.

RECEPTOR: A sensory nerve ending that responds to a stimulus.

RESPITE CARE: The short-term care and supervision of a person with Parkinson's so that his or her care partner can take a break. This care may be provided in the home or in a facility with a respite care program.

RESTING TREMOR: Shaking that occurs in a relaxed and supported limb.

RESTLESS LEGS SYNDROME (RLS): Physical condition marked by an overwhelming urge to move one's legs because of feelings of discomfort. Often happens at night. Can cause legs to jerk and twitch involuntarily.

RETROPULSIVE GAIT: Walking that is propelled backward.

RIGIDITY: A state of stiffness or inflexibility that, in Parkinson's disease, affects the muscles. It is characterized by a constant, even resistance to passive manipulation of the limbs.

ROTENONE: A plant-based pesticide that has been shown to induce Parkinson-like symptoms in laboratory animals.

SEBORRHEA: Increased discharge of the oily secretion sebum from the sebaceous glands of the skin.

SEBORRHOEIC DERMATITIS: Inflammation of the skin sometimes associated with seborrhea.

SEROTONIN: A neurotransmitter that is involved in the control of smooth muscles and nerve impulses, as well as sleep, memory, and mood.

SELECTIVE SEROTONIN REUPTAKE INHIBITORS (SSRIs): A group of antidepressant medications that control serotonin levels in the brain. These drugs are used to treat depression, obsessive-compulsive disorder, panic attacks, and other mood disorders.

SHY-DRAGER SYNDROME: A rare form of parkinsonism in which the symptoms are the result of abnormalities in motor function and problems in the autonomic nervous system. A person with Shy-Drager syndrome has parkinsonism, extremely low blood pressure that worsens upon standing, bladder problems, severe constipation, and decreased sweating. It is one of the Parkinson's Plus syndromes.

SIDE EFFECT: An unintended consequence of a substance or action.

SINEMET: Trade name for the antiparkinson drug that is a mixture of levodopa and carbidopa. This drug combination contains a ratio of levodopa 4 mg or 10 mg to carbidopa 1 mg (Sinemet 100/25, Sinemet 250/25).

SINEMET CR: Controlled-release Sinemet; 200 mg levodopa with 50 mg carbidopa in a capsule contained in a matrix (outer layer) releasing the drug more slowly in the body. These capsules are not to be taken all at once, but rather in separate doses over the course of a day.

SINGLE PHOTON EMISSION COMPUTED TOMOGRAPHY SCAN (SPECT SCAN): An imaging technology similar to a PET scan. It was developed in the 1990s.

STEREOTACTIC SURGERY: Surgical technique that involves placing a small electrode in an area of the brain to destroy a tiny amount of brain tissue.

STRIATONIGRAL DEGENERATION: This is a degeneration of the nerve pathways traveling from the striatum to the substantia nigra. People with this degeneration also appear to have parkinsonism. However, they respond differently to drug therapy than people with Parkinson's.

SUBSTANTIA NIGRA: The black pigmented area of the midbrain where cells manufacture the neurotransmitter dopamine.

SYMMETREL (AMANTADINE): A drug developed to prevent influenza that has been found to control dyskinesia. It may also prescribed as a monotherapy in early Parkinson's disease to treat bradykinesia, rigidity, and tremors.

SYMPATHETIC NERVOUS SYSTEM: The part of the autonomic nervous system originating in the thoracic and lumbar regions of the spinal cord that in general inhibits or opposes the physiological effects of the parasympathetic nervous system, as in tending to reduce digestive secretions or speed up the heart.

THALAMOTOMY: Surgical procedure performed on the brain, in which a small region of the thalamus is destroyed, achieved by stereotactic techniques. Tremor and rigidity in parkinsonism and other conditions may be relieved by thalamotomy.

THALAMUS: Anatomical term designating a mass of gray matter centrally placed deep in the brain near its base and serving as a major relay station for impulses traveling from the spinal cord and cerebellum to the cerebral cortex.

TOXIN: A poisonous substance.

TREMOR: Rhythmic shaking and involuntary movement of part(s) of the body as a result of sequential muscle contractions.

UBIQUITIN CARBOXY-TERMINAL HYDROLASE L1 (UCHL1): Gene suspected in some cases of Parkinson's disease that may be due to heredity.

UNILATERAL: Occurring on one side of the body. Parkinson's symptoms usually begin unilaterally.

"WEARING-OFF" PHENOMENON: Waning of the effect of the last dose of levodopa, associated with abrupt reduction or loss of mobility.

WILSON'S DISEASE: A hereditary disease caused by accumulation of copper in body tissues with neurological symptoms similar to those found in Parkinson's disease.

YOUNG-ONSET PARKINSON'S DISEASE (YOPD): Parkinson's disease that is diagnosed before the average age of onset—fifty-five years old. Some neurologists define "young-onset" as occurring before age forty, but this is arbitrary.

Glossary adapted from the Northwest Parkinson's Foundation, with permission

Resources

Day 1

NATIONAL PARKINSON'S ORGANIZATIONS

(for information, physician contacts or referrals, support group information, speakers, educational materials, etc.)

American Parkinson's Disease Association
1250 Hylan Boulevard, Suite 4B
Staten Island, NY 10305 1946
Phone: 800–223–2732 (in California: 800–908–2372) or
718–981–8001
Fax: 718–981–4399
E-mail: apda@apdapdaparkinson.org
Web: www.apdaparkinson.org

Michael J. Fox Foundation for Parkinson's Research
Grand Central Station
PO Box 4777
New York, NY 10163
Phone: 212–509–0995
Web: www.michaeljfox.org

National Parkinson's Foundation
1501 9th Avenue
Bob Hope Road
Miami, FL 33136–1494
Phone: 800–327–4545 (in Florida: 800–433–7022) or 305–243–6666
Fax: 305–243–5595
E-mail: mailbox@parkinson.org
Web: www.parkinson.org (Web site has "Ask the Doctor," "Ask the Nurse," "Ask the Dietician" features)

Parkinson's Action Network
1025 Vermont Avenue Northwest, Suite 1120
Washington, DC 20005
Phone: 800–850–4726 or 202–842–4101 (California office: 707–544–1994)
E-mail: info@parkinsonsaction.org
Web: www.parkinsonsaction.org

Parkinson's Disease Foundation
710 West 168th Street
New York, NY 10032–9982
Phone: 800–457–6676 or 212–923–4700
Fax: 212–923–4778
E-mail: info@parkinsons-foundation.org
Web: www.pdf.org

Parkinson's Institute
1170 Morse Avenue
Sunnyvale, CA 94089–2958
Phone: 800–786–2958 or 408–734–2800
Fax: 308–734–8522
E-mail: outreach@parkinsonsinstitute.org
Web: www.parkinsonsinstitute.org

Worldwide Education & Awareness for Movement Disorders (WE MOVE)
204 West 84th Street
New York, NY 10024
Phone: 800–437-MOV2 (6682) or 212–875–8312
Fax: 212–875–8289
E-mail: wemove@wemove.org
Web: www.wemove.org

INTERNATIONAL PD ORGANIZATIONS
European Parkinson's Disease Association
www.parkinsonpoly.com/html/en/index.html

OTHER SITES FOR GENERAL PD INFO
ParkinsonsHealth.com
This Web site was created by the pharmaceutical company Teva Neurosciences. It contains information for people who have Parkinson's disease or are concerned that they might, and for care partners. It is written in straightforward, nontechnical language. Web site: www.parkinsonshealth.com

Day 2

Holistic Online
There is an excellent explanation of how Parkinson's disease impacts the dopamine system at this Web site. www.holistic-online.com/Remedies/Parkinson/pd_brain.htm/

Day 3

State-by-State, Plan-by-Plan List of Pharmacy Assistance Programs
Compiled in 2004 by the Association for the Advancement of Retired Persons (AARP)
www.aarp.org/bulletin/prescription/Articles/statebystate.html

Medication Manufacturers' Indigent Drug Program
This Web site lists drug companies that have programs to assist people who cannot afford medications. The list includes companies that produce other medicines in addition to those that treat PD.
Web site: www.parkinsonswellness.org/indigent.html

Boehringer-Ingelheim
The manufacturer of Mirapex has an assistance program. Visit http://us.boehringer-ingelheim.com/about/philanthropy/Patient_Assistance_Program.html or call 1–800–556–8317.

Day 5

National Mental Health Association
Their Web site includes a "therapist finder"—type in your zip code to find a psychiatrist, psychologist, counselor, or social worker in your area. It also has a lot of free information on depression, mental-health advocacy, and resources.
Web site: www.nmha.org

National Institutes of Mental Health
This division of the National Institutes of Health conducts research and produces educational materials on mental health and cognitive effects.
Web site: www.nimh.nih.gov

American Board of Psychiatry and Neurology
For information about neurologists and psychiatrists who have been certified by the American Board of Psychiatry and Neurology, call (847) 945–7900 or visit the group's Web site: www.abpn.com

American Academy of Neurology
1080 Montreal Avenue
Saint Paul, MN 55116
Tel: 800–879–1960 or 651–695–2717
Fax: 651–695–2791
Web site: www.aan.com/public/find.cfm

ORGANIZATIONS AND WEB SITES BY AND FOR PEOPLE WITH PARKINSON'S DISEASE

Clognition.org contains
Web site: www.clognition.org
Grassroots Connection
E-mail: grassrootsconnection@yahoo.com
Web site: http://grassrootsconnection.com
This Web site tracks grassroots PD advocacy and provides information on the latest opportunities to take action. You will also find inspirational success stories of advocates who have Parkinson's or who care for someone who has the disease.

People Living With Parkinson's (PLWP)
Web site: www.PLWP.org
PLWP is a group of individuals with PD who have created an excellent multipurpose Web site that includes a library, a chat room, writing and artwork by people with Parkinson's, personal stories, and much more.

Parkinson's Pipeline Project
Web site: www.pdpipeline.org/index.htm/
This organization is comprised of people with Parkinson's whose aim is to involve patients in the research and development of PD treatments and to speed up the timeline for availability of those treatments. For more information, use the online contact form.

Parkinson's Association of Louisiana (P.A.L.)
P.O. Box 10303
New Orleans, LA 70101–0303
2030 Dickory Avenue, Suite 202
Hanrahan, LA 70123
Phone: 504–733–7203
Web site: www.parkinsonla.org
P.A.L. provides support, education, and funding for people in Louisiana who are affected by Parkinson's disease. A variety of merchandise for raising awareness of PD (bracelets, pins, ribbons) can be purchased from the organization, too.

Texas Parkinson's Action Network
"Travels With Parkinson's" Internet radio show
Web site: http://pwnkle.com/travels/index.htm
The program is hosted by Leonard "Chy" [pronounced "Shy"] Casavant. Chy has Parkinson's disease and interviews interesting Parkies from around the world.

Young-Onset Parkinson's Association (YOPA)
Phone: 866–869–9672
Web site: www.yopa.org
This organization is for young people with PD.

YoungParkinsons.com
This Web site is for younger people with PD. It offers a variety of services, including a daily PD news feature, chat room, PD awareness merchandise, personal stories, information centers on issues like stem cells, deep-brain stimulation, and PET scans as diagnostic tools.

Regional/smaller organizations

HollyRod Foundation
9250 Wilshire Boulevard, Suite 220
Beverly Hills, CA 90212
Phone: 866-HOLLYROD (866-465-5976)
Fax: 310-385-1599
E-mail: info@hollyrod.com

Muhammad Ali Parkinson's Research Center Disease Registry
The comprehensive Parkinson's disease registry that has been developed by the
Muhammad Ali Parkinson Research Center in Phoenix, Arizona, collects information
about all sorts of chemical exposures, head injuries, and other experiences that may be
linked to PD.
Web site: www.maprc.com/home/info/registry.aspx

Northwest Parkinson's Foundation
Bill Bell, Executive Director
PO Box 56
Mercer Island, WA 98040
Phone: 877-980-7500
E-mail: nwpf@nwpf.org
Web site: www.nwpf.org
NWPF has a free weekly electronic newsletter that is an excellent source of information
on the latest resources, events, and personal stories. You can subscribe by sending an e-
mail to nwpf@nwpf.org.

Week 2

Source of CoQ10 used in Archives of Neurology study:
Vitaline Corporation (www.vitalinecoq10.com)

The ParkinsonPoly Web site (www.parkinsonpoly.com/html/en/therapy/exercise-
role.html) has a free online video that can be downloaded to your computer. The video
demonstrates exercises that are specifically for people with PD.

Also helpful: *Parkinson's Disease and the Art of Moving*, book and DVD, by John
Argue, issued by New Harbinger Publications (February 15, 2000). ISBN 1572241837.
Available at large bookstores.

Week 3

National Family Caregivers Association
Web site: www.nfcacares.org

Children of Aging Parents (CAPS)
PO Box 167
Richboro, PA 18954
Phone: 800-227-7294
Web site: www.caps4caregivers.org

Family Caregiver Alliance (FCA)
180 Montgomery Street, Ste 1100
San Francisco, CA 94104
Phone: 415–434–3388 or 800–445–8106
Fax: 415–434–3508
E-mail: info@caregiver.org
Web site: www.caregiver.org

Aging Parents and Elder Care
Web site: www.aging-parents-and-elder-care.com
Their site has many helpful fact sheets.

National Organization for Empowering Caregivers
Web sites: www.nofec.org and www.care-givers.com
This site has an extensive list of resources for care partners, ranging from respite-care
contacts to online chat rooms and support groups to social service agencies.

BenefitsCheckup.org—a project of the National Council on Aging
Web site: www.benefitscheckup.org
"BenefitsCheckUp helps thousands every day to find programs for people ages 55 and
over that may pay for some of their costs of prescription drugs, health-care, utilities, and
other essential items or services."

APTA Neurology Section
PO Box 327
Alexandria, VA 22313
Phone: 1–800–999–2782, ext. 8588
Fax: 703–706–8578
E-mail: neuropta.org
Web site: www.neuropt.org/consumers/resrcindx.cfm
Neurology section of the American Physical Therapy Association

The American Occupational Therapy Association
4720 Montgomery Lane—PO Box 31220
Bethesda, MD 20824–1220
Phone: 301–652–2682, TDD: 800–377–8555
Fax: 301–652–7711
Web site: www.aota.org/
Contacts for state occupational therapy associations:
www.aota.org/featured/area6/links/LINK03.asp

Caregivers Marketplace
Web site: www.caregiversmarketplace.com
The Caregivers Marketplace can meet all sorts of needs that care partners may have,
whether it is information, links to other resources, discounts on adaptive equipment and
products, and a "cash back" program.

Home Accessibility Funding Resources Guide, produced by the Minnesota Housing
Finance Agency
www.mhfa.state.mn.us/homes/Access_Financing_Grid.pdf. The online copy of this guide
covers many federal resources for grants and low-interest loan programs if you need to
remodel your home to make it accessible. Also includes links to federal income-tax
information.

Guide to Buying a Home for People with Disabilities: Accessible Homes and Accessible Home Modifications by New Horizons Un-Limited, Inc., published January 2, 2002 [Revised April 30, 2002]
Guide can be found at: www.new-horizons.org/gdbhac.html

Links to individual state offices of Centers for Independent Living
Web site: www.new-horizons.org/indcil.html

Week 4

Caregiving.com
Web site: www.caregiving.com
Caregiving.com has online support groups for care partners.

NIMH
The complete NIMH fact sheet, "Depression and Parkinson's Disease" is available at www.nimh.nih.gov/publicat/depparkinson.cfm/.

SharetheCare.org
"Share the Care: How to Organize a Group to Care for Someone Who is Seriously Ill" is available from www.sharethecare.org.

Month 2

Enablemart:
Toll-Free: 888-640-1999, outside the U.S.: 360-695-4155
Fax: 360-695-4133
Web site: www.enablemart.com/default.aspx?store=16
Vendor of adaptive technology; call for a catalog

RehabTool.com
Web site: www.rehabtool.com/at.html

Month 3

National Respite Coalition
4016 Oxford Street
Annandale, VA, 22003
Contact: Jill Kagan
Phone: 1-703-256-9578
E-mail: jbkaganol.com

National Respite Locator Service
Web site: www.respitelocator.org/index.htm

National Association for Home Care
228 7th Street, SE
Washington, DC 20003
Phone: 202–547–7424
Fax: 202–547–3540
This organization is comprised of providers of home care and hospice service. Their Web site has a search feature to help you to find providers in your area.
Web site: www.nahc.org

National Center for Biotechnology Information
Web site: www.ncbi.nlm.nih.gov/gquery/gquery.fcgi. This agency has an amazing meta-search engine that searches many government databases at once for relevant agencies.

Month 10

Aptiva site by Medtronic
www.newhopeforparkinsons.org
Information about deep-brain stimulation

DBS-STN.org
Web site: www.dbs-stn.org
This site is an affiliate of the Parkinson's Alliance and is intended for people with PD who have had or are contemplating deep brain stimulation (DBS) surgery. It contains the latest research on DBS, information on support services for DBS patients, an online forum to discuss experiences, and personal stories from people who have had this surgery to treat their PD.

Month 11

CLINICAL TRIALS

- Acurian: www.acurian.com
- National Institutes of Health (NIH): www.nih.gov or www.clinical trials.gov
- National Institute of Neurological Diseases and Stroke (NINDS): www.ninds.nih.gov or www.clinicaltrials.com
- PDtrials.org: www.PDtrials.org
- Veritas Medicine: www.veritasmedicine.com

Morris K. Udall Centers of Excellence

- Brigham & Women's Hospital, Boston, MA. Director: Peter Lansbury, Jr., PhD: http://www.ninds.nih.gov/funding/research/parkinsons web/udall_centers/brigham.htm
- Columbia University, New York, NY. Director: Robert Burke, MD: http://www.ninds.nih.gov/funding/research/parkinsonsweb/udall_centers/columbia.htm
- Harvard University/McLean Hospital, Boston, MA. Director: Ole Isacson, MD: http://www.ninds.nih.gov/funding/research/parkinsons web/udall_centers/harvard.htm
- Johns Hopkins University, Baltimore, MD. Director: Ted M. Dawson, MD, PhD: www.ninds.nih.gov/funding/research/parkinsonsweb/udall_centers/hopkins.htm
- Massachusetts General Hospital/Massachusetts Institute of Technology, Boston, MA. Director: Anne Young, MD, PhD: http://www.ninds.nih.gov/funding/research/parkinsonsweb/udall_centers/mit.htm
- Mayo Clinic, Jacksonville, FL. Director: Dennis W. Dickson, MD: http://www.ninds.nih.gov/funding/research/parkinsonsweb/udall_centers/mayo.htm
- Northwestern University, Evanston, IL. Director: D. James Surmeier, MD.
- University of California–Los Angeles, Los Angeles, CA. Director: Marie-Francoise S. Chesselet, MD: http://www.ninds.nih.gov/funding/research/parkinsonsweb/udall_centers/ucla.htm
- University of Kentucky Medical Center, Lexington, KY. Director: Greg A. Gerhardt, PhD: http://www.ninds.nih.gov/funding/research/parkinsonsweb/udall_centers/kentucky.htm
- University of Pittsburgh, Pittsburgh, PA. Director: Michael J. Zigmond, MD: http://www.ninds.nih.gov/funding/research/parkinsons web/udall_centers/pittsburgh.htm
- University of Virginia, Charlottesville, VA. Director: G. Fred Wooten, MD: http://www.ninds.nih.gov/funding/research/parkinsonsweb/udall_centers/uva.htm

AMERICAN PARKINSON'S DISEASE ASSOCIATION ADVANCED CENTERS

- ○ Boston University School of Medicine, Boston, MA
- ○ Emory University School of Medicine, Atlanta, GA
- ○ Massachusetts General Hospital, Boston, MA
- ○ UCLA School of Medicine, Los Angeles, CA
- ○ UMDNJ Robert Wood Johnson Medical School, New Brunswick, NJ
- ○ University of Virginia Medical Center, Charlottesville, VA
- ○ Washington University Medical Center, St. Louis, MO

NATIONAL PARKINSON FOUNDATION CENTERS OF EXCELLENCE

Arizona
Muhammad Ali Parkinson Research Center
Barrow Neurological Institute
500 W Thomas Road, Suite 720
Phoenix, AZ 85013
Contact: Margaret Anne Coles
Phone: 602–406–4931
E-mail: mcles@chw.edu
Web site: www.maprc.com

California
The California Neuroscience Institute at St. John's Regional Medical Center—NPF
Center of Excellence
1700 N. Rose Avenue, Ste 400
Oxnard, CA 93030
Contact: Susan Kline
Phone: 805–988–7599
E-mail: skline@chw.edu
Web site: stjohnshealth.org

The Parkinson's Disease and Other Movement Disorders Center
The Keck School of Medicine, Dept. of Neurology, University of Southern California
1510 San Pablo Street, HCC Suite 268
Los Angeles, CA 90033–4606
Contact: Carol Corser
Phone: 323–442–6206
E-mail: ccorser@surgery.usc.edu
Web site: www.usc.edu

University of California–San Francisco Parkinson's Disease Clinic and Research Center
503 Parnassus Avenue, Room M-348
San Francisco, CA 94143–0216
Contact: Mariann DiMinno
Phone: 415–476–9276
E-mail: mdm30@itsa.ucsf.edu

Colorado
Colorado Neurological Institute—Movement Disorders Center
701 East Hampden Avenue, Suite 530
Englewood, CO 80113
Contact: Josette Pressler
Phone: 303–762–6679
E-mail: pressler@megapathdsl.net
Web site: www.theCNI.org

Florida
University of Florida McKnight Brain Institute—NPF Clinical Center
100 S. Newell Drive, Room L3–100
Gainesville, FL 32610
Contact: Sarah Munson
Phone: 404–728–4957
E mail: munsos@neurology.ufl.edu
Web site: www.ufbi.ufl.edu

Georgia
Medical College of Georgia
4 South Nursing Unit
Augusta, GA 30912
Contact: Caroline diDonato
Phone: 706–721–2798
E-mail: cdidonato@mail.mcg.edu
Web site: www.mcg.edu

Illinois
Alexian Neurosciences Institute
1786 Moon Lake Boulevard
Hoffman Estates, IL 60194
Contact: Paula Wiener
Phone: 888–365–5240
E-mail: paula.wienerbbhh.net
Web site: www.alexian-neurosciences.org

Northwestern University Parkinson's Disease & Movement Disorders Center—NPF
Center of Excellence
710 North Lakeshore Drive
11th Floor, Abbot Hall
Chicago, IL 60611
Contact: Diane Breslow
Phone: 312–503–2970
E-mail: dbreslow@nmff.org
Web site: www.parkinsons.northwestern.edu

Southern Illinois University School of Medicine
Department of Neurology
751 N. Rutledge
Springfield, IL 62794–9643
Contact: Charlene Young
Phone: 217–545–7209
E-mail: cyoung@siumed.edu

Kansas
University of Kansas Med Ctr Research
Institute Inc
Kansas City, KS 66160–0001
Contact: Rajesh Pahwa
Phone: 913–588–6970
Web site: www.kumc.edu/parkinson

Maryland
Johns Hopkins Parkinson's Disease and Movement Disorders Center
Johns Hopkins Outpatient Center (JHOC)
601 N Caroline Street, Suite 5064
Baltimore, MD 21287
Contact: Becky Dunlop
Phone: 410–955–8795
E-mail: rdunlop@jhmi.edu
Web site: www.neuro.jhmi.edu/hopkinspdmd

Massachusetts
Massachusetts General Hospital, Harvard Medical School—NPF Center of Excellence
32 Fruit Street
Boston, MA 02114
Contact: Anne Young, MD, PhD
Phone: 617–726–2383

Michigan
Clinical Neuroscience Center
William Beaumont Hospital
26400 W. Twelve Mile Road, Suite 110
Southfield, MI 48034
Contact: Dawn Miller
Phone: (248) 352–8628

Minnesota
Struthers Parkinson's Center
6701 Country Club Drive
Golden Valley, MN 55427
Contact: Joan Gardner
Phone: 952–993–5495
E-mail: gardnj@parknicollet.com

New York

The Betty and Morton Yarmon Center for Parkinson's Disease at Beth Israel
MedicalCenter—NPF Center of Excellence
10 Union Square East
Suite 2R
New York, NY 10003
Contact: Karyn Boyar
E-mail: kboyar@chpnet.org
Phone: 212–844–8379

Kings County Hospital
450 Clarkson Avenue #1213
Brooklyn, NY 11203–2056
Contact: Olie Westheimer
Phone: 718–270–4232
E-mail: westheimer@sprynet.com

University of Rochester Medical Center
Department of Neurology
919 Westfall Road, C-220
Rochester, NY 14618
Contact: Irenita Gardiner
Phone: 585–341–7569
E-mail: nita.gardinercc.rochester.edu

North Carolina

University of North Carolina at Chapel Hill School of Medicine
Dept. of Neurology
CB 7025, 3114 Bioinformatics Bldg.
Chapel Hill, NC 27599–7025
Contact: Nancy Kosanovich, NP
Phone: 919–966–5549
E-mail: kosanovn@neurology.unc.edu
Web site: nerve.neurology.unc.edu/neurology/

Ohio

Center for Neurological Restoration, Cleveland Clinic Foundation
S31, 9500 Euclid Avenue
Cleveland, OH 44195
Contact: Monique Giroux
Phone: 216–444–8001

Madden/NPF Center of Excellence for Parkinson's Disease and Related Movement
Disorders, The Ohio State University
371 McCampbell Hall
1581 Dodd Drive
Columbus, OH 43210–1128
Contact: Angela Campbell
Phone: 614–292–8607
E-mail: campbell-9@medctr.osu.edu
Web site: www.neurology.med.ohio-state.edu/movementdisorders/

Oregon
Oregon Health & Science University
3181 SW Sam Jackson Park Road
Portland, OR 97239–3079
Contact: Lisa Mann, RN, BSN
Phone: 503–494–7230
E-mail: mannli@ohsu.edu
Web site: www.ohsu.edu/pco

Pennsylvania
Parkinson's Disease and Movement Disorders Center of the University of Pennsylvania
330 South Ninth Street, 2nd Floor
Philadelphia, PA 19107
Contact: Suzanne Reichwein
Phone: 215–829–7273
E-mail: sreichwein@pahosp.com
Web site: www.pennhealth.com

University of Pittsburgh
3471 5th Avenue
Suite 810
Pittsburgh, PA 15213–3583
Contact: Rita Vareha
Phone: 412–692–4916
E-mail: rav9@pitt.edu

Tennessee
Vanderbilt University Med Cntr.
C-3321 Mecial Center N
Nashville, TN 37212
Contact: Ariel Deutch, PhD
Phone: 615–936–0060
E-mail: ariel.deutch@vanderbilt.edu
Web site: www.mc.vanderbilt.edu/deutchlab/npf.htm

Texas
Parkinson's Disease Center & Movement Disorders Clinic at Baylor College of Medicine—NPF Center of Excellence
6550 Fannin Street
Suite 1801
Houston, TX 77030
Contact: Christine Hunter
Phone: 713–798–7438
E-mail: neurons@bcm.tmc.edu

Scott & White Clinic, Texas A & M University Health Science Center—NPF Center of Excellence
TX A&M Univ. Health Science Center, College of Medicine
2401 South 31st Street
Temple, TX 76508
Contact: Patricia Simpson
Phone: 254–724–2465
E-mail: psimpson@swmail.sw.org

Wisconsin
Aurora Sinai Medical Center—NPF Center of Excellence
Wisconsin Parkinson Association
945 N 12 Street, Suite 4602
Milwaukee, WI 53233
Contact: Henrietta Riley
Phone: 800–972–5455
E-mail: Gloria.Bockurora.org
Web site: www.wiparkinson.org

Month 11

Insurance for Dummies by Jack Hungelmann
ISBN 0764552945
Jack has been an insurance agent for more than twenty-five years and used this experience to assemble a book that is useful to any consumer, but is particularly helpful to someone with a chronic illness.

Long-Term Care Insurance National Advisory Council
Web site: www.longtermcareinsurance.org

Bibliography

Ali, Ahmed S., MD, and John E. Morley, MD. "Treatment of Parkinson's Disease (PD)." Cyberounds InterMDnet, http://www.cyberounds.com/conf/geriatrics/1999–02–05/index.html.

Amgen, Inc. "Following Complete Review of Phase 2 Trial Data Amgen Confirms Decision to Halt GDNF Study; Comprehensive Review of Scientific Findings, Patient Safety, Drove Decision." *Business Wire* (February 11, 2005).

Bower, J. H., MD, D. M. Maraganore, MD, B. J. Peterson, BS, S. K. McDonnell, MS, J. E. Ahlskog, PhD, MD, and W. A. Rocca, MD, MPH. "Head Trauma Preceding PD: A Case-Control Study." *Neurology* 60 (2003): 1610–15.

Cannuscio, C. C., C. Jones, I. Kawachi, G. A. Colditz, L. Berkman, and E. Rimm. "Reverberation of Family Illness: A Longitudinal Assessment of Informal Caregiver and Mental Health Status in the Nurses' Health Study." *American Journal of Public Health* 92 (2002):305–1311

Cerner Multum, Inc. "Tasmar." Version 1.07 (January 23, 2004). Drug Information Online Web site, www.drugs.com.

_____. "Selegiline." Version 3.06 (revision September 9, 2004). Drug Information Online Web site, www.drugs.com.

Chen, Jack J., PharmD, BCPS, CGP. "Neuroprotection in Parkinson's Disease." American College of Clinical Pharmacy Annual Meeting, November 2–5, 2003, Atlanta, Georgia. http://www.medscape.com/viewarticle/467106_4 (posted January 20, 2004).

Chong S. Lee, MD, FRCPC. "Levodopa-Induced Dyskinesia: Mechanisms and Management." *British Columbia Medical Journal* 43, no. 4 (May 2001): 206–09. http://www.bcma.org/public/bc_medical_journal/BCMJ/2001/may_2001/PDDyskinesia.asp.

"ConsumerLab.com Finds Discrepancies in Strength of CoQ10 Supplements." *Townsend Letter for Doctors and Patients* (August–September 2004).

Cram, David L., MD. *Understanding Parkinson's Disease: A Self-Help Guide*. Omaha: Addicus Books, 2001), 54.

Cummings, J. "A Window on the Role of Dopamine in Addiction Disorders." *Journal of Neurology, Neurosurgery and Psychiatry* 68 (April 2000): 404 http://jnnp.bmjjournals.com/cgi/content/full/68/4/404.

"The Different Types of Massage Therapy." http://www.trinbagoinfo.com/mta/association/typesofmassagetherapy.htm.

Di Minno, Mariann, RN, MA, and Michael J. Aminoff, MD, DSc. "Parkinson Primer." National Parkinson Foundation Web site (www.parkinson.org).

_____ . Treatment Options, National Parkinson Foundation Web site (www.parkinson.org).

Greenamyre, J. Timothy and Teresa G. Hastings. "Parkinson's—Divergent Causes, Convergent Mechanisms." *Science* 304, no. 5,674 (May 21, 2004), 1120–22, http://www.sciencemag.org/cgi/content/full/304/5674/1120#ref3.

Gschwandtner, Ute, Jacqueline Aston, Susanne Renaud, and Peter Fuhr. "Pathologic Gambling in Patients with Parkinson's Disease." *Clinical Neuropharmacology* 24 , no. 3 (May/June 2001):170–72.

Holden, Kathrynne, MS, RD. "Fava Beans, Levodopa and Parkinson's Disease." (2001) National Parkinson Foundation Web site, www.parkinson.org/.

_____."Parkinson's, B6, B12, and Folate: What's the Connection?" *Parkinson Report: Official Journal of the National Parkinson Foundation* 13, no. 2 (Spring-Summer 2002):8–10.

"How Does an MRI Work?" www.msu.edu/~gallard1/4.htm.

Hubble, Jean Pintar, MD and Richard C. Bertou. *Parkinson's Disease: Medications*. Miami: National Parkinson Foundation, Inc., 1996–99.

Hungelmann, Jack. "What Young-Onset Persons with Parkinson's and Caregivers Need to Know about Insurance and Insurance-Related Government Programs." *Parkinson Report: Official Journal of the National Parkinson Foundation* 16, no. 2 (Spring 2005):21–26.

———. *Insurance for Dummies*. Hoboken, NJ: John Wiley & Sons, 2001.

Institute of Medicine of the National Academies, *Dietary Reference Intakes: Vitamins* (2001) http://www.iom.edu/Object.File/Master/7/296/0.pdf/.

Ives, Jeffrey C., PhD, and Jacob Sosnoff, "Beyond the Mind-Body Exercise Hype." *The Physician and Sportsmedicine* 28, no. 3 (March 2000).

Jahanshahi, Marjan, and C. David Marsden. *Parkinson's Disease: A Self-Help Guide for Patients and Their Families*. London: Souvenir Press, 1998.

Jankovic, Joseph, MD. "What is the role of CoQ10 in the treatment of Parkinson's disease (PD)?" Baylor College of Medicine Department of Neurology, http://www.bcm.edu/neurology/struct/parkinson/coq10.html (modified March 3, 2005).

Kaasinen, V, E. Nurmi, J. Bergman, O. Eskola, O, Solin, P, Sonninen, and J. O. Rinne. "Personality Traits and Brain Dopaminergic Function in Parkinson's disease." *Proceedings of the National Academy of Sciences USA* 98, no. 23 (November 6, 2001): 13,272–77.

Kontakos, Natalie, and Julie Stokes. "Monograph Series on Aging-related Diseases: XII. Parkinson's Disease—Recent Developments and New Directions." *Chronic Diseases in Canada* 20 (2003): 58-76.

Körner, Yvonne, Charlotte Meindorfner, Jens Carsten Möller, Karin Stiasny-Kolster, Doris Haja, Werner Cassel, Wolfgang Hermann Oertel, and Hans-Peter Krüger. "Predictors of Sudden Onset of Sleep in Parkinson's Disease. *Movement Disorders* 19, no. 11 (2004): 1298–305.

Kübler-Ross, Elisabeth, MD. *On Death and Dying*. Scribner Classics, January 1997.

Lai, Benjamin C. L., MD, MSc, and Joseph K. C. Tsui, MD, FRCP (UK), FRCPC. "Epidemiology of Parkinson's Disease." *BC Medical Journal* (British Columbia) 43, no. 3 (2001): 133–37.

Langston, J. William. "Accelerating Research on Genes and Environment in Parkinson's Disease." *Environmental Health Perspectives: 128 Essays on the Future of Environmental Health Research*. http://ehp.niehs.nih.gov/docs/2005/7937/7937.htm.

Langston J. W., P. Ballard, J. W. Tetrud, and I. Irwin. "Chronic Parkinsonism in Humans Due to a Product of Meperidine-Analog Synthesis." *Science* 219, no. 4587 (February 25, 1983): 979–80.

Leader, Geoffrey, MD and and Lucille Leader. *Parkinson's Disease: The Way Forward! An Integrated Approach including Drugs, Surgery, Nutrition, Bowel and Muscle Function, Self-Esteem, Sexuality, Stress Control and Carers.* London: Denor Press, 2001.

Lee Silverman Voice Treatment, LSVT Foundation web site, http://www.lsvt.org/main_site.htm

Lieberman, Abraham, MD. "Parkinson Disease, Parkinson-Like, Parkinson-Plus, Atypical Parkinson Disease, Parkinson Syndrome, Parkinsonism." National Parkinson Foundation Web site. www.parkinson.org (April 1, 2002.)

_____. *Shaking Up Your Doctor: Getting the Most from Your Visit.* Miami: National Parkinson Foundation, 2002.

_____. *Shaking Up Parkinson's Disease: Fighting Like a Tiger, Thinking Like a Fox.* Sudbury, MA: Jones and Bartlett, 2002.

_____. "What You Should Know About Young-Onset Parkinson Disease (YOPD) and Other Parkinson-like Diseases that Appear below Age 40 Years" (March 29, 2004). National Parkinson Foundation Web site, www.parkinson.org

Liu, Bin, Hui-Ming Gao, and Jau-Shyong Hong. "Parkinson's Disease and Exposure to Infectious Agents and Pesticides and the Occurrence of Brain Injuries: Role of Neuroinflammation." *Environmental Health Perspectives* 111, no. 8 (June 2003).

Marjama-Lyons, Jill, MD. and Mary J. Shomon. *What Your Doctor May Not Tell You about Parkinson's Disease: A Holistic Program for Optimal Wellness.* New York: Warner Books, 2003.

Marsh, Laura, MD, and Ariel Berk. "Neuropsychiatric Aspects of Parkinson's Disease: Recent Advances." *Current Psychiatry Reports* 5.

Mayo Clinic–Jacksonville, Florida. "Mayo Clinic Researchers and Former Colleagues Find Cause of Family's Parkinson's Disease." *Mayo Clinic Checkup Newsletter* 10, no. 4 (December 2003).

Mayo Clinic staff. "Dementia: Not Always Alzheimer's" (March 7, 2005). www.mayoclinic.com

Medtronic, Inc., "Questions and Answers about Activa Parkinson's Control Therapy." www.medtronic.com/neuro/parkinsons/activa_qa4.html. Version 1.04, updated May 1, 2004.

Merino, Jose G., MD, Jose Luchsinger, MD, MPH, and Zhigao Huang, MD, PhD. "Parkinson's Disease Dementia." www.emedicine.com/med/topic3110.htm (October 13, 2004).

Michael J. Fox Foundation for Parkinson's Research. "The Michael J. Fox Foundation for Parkinson's Research to Fund Research for Parkinson's Biomarker" (April 10, 2002). Michael J. Fox Foundation for Parkinson's Research Web site. www.michaeljfox.org.

_____. "New Test May Detect Parkinson's Early, Aid Search for Drugs" (accessed January 5, 2005). Michael J. Fox Foundation for Parkinson's Research, http://www.michaeljfox.org/news/article.php?id=143&sec=4.

Moyer, Paula, MA. "Ibuprofen May Protect Against Parkinson's Disease." Medscape Medical News. www.medscape.com/viewarticle/503152/ (April 14, 2005).

Myers, John Peterson, PhD. "Gene Expression and Environmental Exposures: New Opportunities for Disease Prevention." *San Francisco Medicine*, Opinion (April 15, 2004).

National Institute of Environmental Health Sciences, "Role of the Environment in Parkinson's Disease" (revised April 14, 2003). http://www.niehs.nih.gov/oc/factsheets/parkinson/home.htm.

National Institute of Neurological Diseases and Stroke and National Institutes of Health. "Parkinson's Disease: Challenges, Progress, and Promise." http://www.ninds.nih.gov/disorders/parkinsons_disease/parkinsons_research.htm (November 2004).

National Institute of Neurological Diseases and Stroke. "Parkinson's Disease: Hope Through Research." National Institute of Neurological Diseases and Stroke, http://www.ninds.nih.gov/disorders/parkinsons_disease/detail_parkinsons_disease.htm (updated May 3, 2005).

National Institute on Aging. "Scientists Detect Probable Genetic Cause of Parkinson's Disease." National Institute on Aging Web site. http://www.nia.nih.gov/NewsAndEvents/PressReleases/PR20040117Parkinsons.htm/.

National Institutes of Mental Health (NIMH). "Depression and Parkinson's Disease." (May 2002) National Institutes of Mental Health Web site. www.nimh.nih.gov/publicat/depparkinson.cfm.

Nausieda, Paul, MD, and Gloria Bock, MSN, RN, CS. *Parkinson's Disease: What You and Your Family Should Know.* Miami: National Parkinson Foundation, 2000.

Neufeld, Shari, MA, CSW. "Coping with Caregiver Burnout." Parkinson's Control.com. http://parkinsonscontrol.com/parkinsons/articles/copecaregiverburnout.asp (December 12, 2002).

Parkinson's Action Network. "What Is Parkinson's Disease?" Parkinson's Action Network. http://www.parkinsonsaction.org/aboutparkinsons/whatisparkinsons .htm (accessed February 23, 2005).

"Parkinson's Disease (Shaking Palsy)." *Merck Manual of Diagnosis and Therapy.* http://www.merck.com/mrkshared/mmanual/section14/chapter179/ 179e.jsp/.

Parkinson's Disease Foundation. *Frequently Asked Questions About Parkinson's Disease.* New York: Parkinson's Disease Foundation, 2004.

Parkinson's Disease Society. "Jane Asher Announces Parkinson's Awareness Week." Parkinson's Disease Society. http://www.parkinsons.org.uk (April 2005).

Parkinson's Pipeline Project. "Amgen Halts GDNF Trial: What's All the Controversy About?" http://www.pdpipeline.org/amgen_gdnf_halt.htm (revised February 22, 2005).

Pfeiffer, Ronald, MD. "Parkinson's Disease and Nonmotor Function." *Parkinson's Report: Official Journal of the National Parkinson Foundation* (April 2005): 3–9.

Poorkaj, Parvoonah, Lina Moses, Jennifer S. Montimurro, John G. Nutt, Gerard D. Schellenberg, and Haydeh Payami. "Parkin Mutation Dosage and the Phenomenon of Anticipation: A Molecular Genetic Study of Familial Parkinsonism." Biomed Central Neurology. *BMC Neurology* 5, no. 4 (2005) doi:10.1186/1471–2377–5-4. Accessed via http://dx.doi.org/.

Saito, Kensen, "The Shiatsu Story," *Canadian College of Shiatsu Therapy, Japan Shiatsu Clinic Newsletter,* http://www.oyayubi.com/newsletter.html#The%20Shiatsu%20Story

Salloway, Stephen D., MD, MS. "Neuropsychiatric Aspects of Movement Disorders." http://www.brown.edu/Departments/Clinical_Neurosciences/ articles/ss54993.html.

Schuster, Larry. "Pessimism, Anxiety Tied to Parkinson's" (April 15, 2005). Reuters Health. www.reutershealth.org.

Sharma, Nutan, MD, and Elaine Richman, PhD. *Parkinson's Disease and the Family: A New Guide.* Cambridge, MA: Harvard University Press, 2005.

Shiatsu Academy of Tokyo. "A Brief History of Shiatsu." http://www.kensensaito .com/history.htm.

Sierpina, Victor S., MD, and Moshe S. Frenkel, MD. "Acupuncture: A Clinical Review." *Southern Medical Journal* 8, no. 3 (2005): 330–37.

Stem Cells: Scientific Progress and Future Research Directions. Department of Health and Human Services. June 2001. http://stemcells.nih.gov/info/scireport, 17.

Stem Cell Institute. "Stem Cell 101." University of Minnesota Stem Cell Institute. www.stemcell.umn.edu/stemcell/stemce11101.html (last modified September 20, 2004).

"Tai Chi and Yohimbine Could Help Parkinson's" (November 13, 2002). Healthline. www.reutershealth.com.

University of Pennsylvania. "Olfactory Function in Relatives of Patients with Parkinson's Disease." PDtrials Web site. www.pdtrials.org/.

U.S. Equal Employment Opportunity Commission, U.S. Department of Justice, Civil Rights Division. "Americans with Disabilities Act/Questions and Answers" (Washington, DC: August 23, 2002). http://ada.gov/q&aeng02.htm.

_____. Facts about the Americans with Disabilities Act (Washington, DC: January 15, 1997). www.eeoc.gov/facts/fs-ada.html.

Waknine, Yael. "Early Rasagiline Therapy Shows Long-Term Benefits for Parkinson's." Medscape Medical News. www.medscape.com/viewarticle/501285 (March 10, 2005).

Welshons, John E. *Awakening from Grief: Finding the Way Back to Joy.* Maui, Hawaii: Inner Ocean Publishing, August 1, 2003.

Worldwide Education and Awareness for Movement Disorders (WE MOVE). "Experimental Therapies." WE MOVE Web site. www.wemove.org/par/par_ethe.html (updated January 19, 2005).

_____. "Overview of Multiple System Atrophy." WE MOVE Web site. www.wemove.org/msa/.

_____. "Overview of Progressive Supranuclear Palsy." WE MOVE Web site. www.wemove.org/psp/.

Acknowledgments

SO MANY people gave me their love and support, their questions and stories, encouragement and inspiration when I took on this project. First of all, thank you to my editor, Sue McCloskey, and Marlowe & Company for offering me this life-changing opportunity.

My husband, Paul, deserves some kind of hazardous-duty bonus for hanging in there during some of my "meltdown" moments when my neck and shoulders were in knots from poor computer posture; crises of confidence; and extreme neglect in household maintenance. Thank you, Alex and Bennett, for sharing your mom with this project, asking questions about PD, letting me talk to your classmates about PD, and for being such wonderful boys. Now that this is done, we can spend much more time together. I still have dibs on the laptop, though. My parents, "Bud" and Rosemary Hunt, and my in-laws, Jack and Marge Christensen, have given me their love, encouragement, and support, as have Annie Shull, Carole Dostal, Carrie Carlson, Louise LeCoque, George Fell, and Reverend Margaret Dostal Fell.

Our close friends Linda Simon, Glenn Olson, Sam and Robert gave me free time for writing by keeping the guys occupied and have opened their hearts, their home and their cabin to us as we deal with this disease. We love you guys!

My "fairy godmother" Terre Thomas has been there with words of wisdom, a willing ear, cinnamon tea for long talks and chakra tea for long soaks in the tub to heal my spirit and my body.

All of the staff at the Institute for Agriculture and Trade Policy in Minneapolis has been full of encouragement and support. Special thanks to Tyson Acker, Candace Falk, Char Greenwald, Kathy Hiltsley, Kate Hoff, Jim Kleinschmit, Marie Kulick, Patti Landres, Ben Lilliston, Ricki McMillan, Mark Ritchie, Niel Ritchie, Kathleen Schuler, David Wallinga, and Lesley White. My environmental health colleagues—Michael Lerner, Pete Myers, Charlotte Brody, Gary Cohen, Ted Schettler, Tracey Easthope, Charlie Cray, Monica Rohde Buckhorn, Laurie Valeriano, Monica Moore, and the late Mary Beth Doyle—have all been inspirational.

My sincere gratitude to Peter Barnes and members of the Mesa Refuge board of directors for providing me with the opportunity of a lifetime, and to Pam Carr, for her exemplary service as caretaker. I will never forget my two weeks at Mesa Refuge and hope to be able to return sometime. Mesa Refuge gave me the solitude and peace that I needed to begin writing.

This book could not have been completed without the help of many people within the Parkinson's community. So many people within the Parkinson's community have touched my life in ways that I believe have helped me to become a better person and to deal better with the disease. Many have been mentioned already but merit it again: Joan Samuelson, Michael J. Fox, Muhammad Ali. Others, such as all of the advocates and state and congressional coordinators, are too numerous to list. My deepest apologies in advance for anyone that I might have missed.

My dear friend Bill Bell offered unwavering encouragement, sage advice, seemingly infinite patience with my frequent outbursts of panic and self-doubt, and his dry sense of humor, which has somehow survived the soggy Pacific Northwest climate.

I have been very fortunate to have Dr. Paul Tuite at the Movement Disorders Center at the University of Minnesota as my physician. He has been a source of information, editorial review, and advice for this book and an advocate for me and his other PD patients. I applaud him and his staff for taking a holistic approach to research and patient care.

Barbara Davidson has been a godsend, volunteering her excellent editing skills and thoughtful comments that added so much to many parts of book. Joanna Glickler of the Northwest Parkinson Foundation and Adolfo Diaz of the National Parkinson Foundation helped with survey distribution. Thanks, too, Joanna, for the tip about SurveyMonkey.

The members of our support group have helped us so much. We love you guys! Hugs to Gene, Anita, Dan and Arlene, Jack and Judy, Deb and Andy, Gary and Mary Ann, Dale and Linda, Bob and Susan, Dave and Katie, and Linda and Wayne.

Parkies and care partners who contributed to the survey or in phone or E-mail conversations included Mike O'Leary, Pam Milton, Jay Adams-Feuer, Kevin Burkart, Michael, Ken Willkomm, Carol Meenen, Marcie, Paula Tomlin, Linda Herman, Paul, Jeannie Lewis, Linda Cooper, Karl and Angela Robb, Joan M. Gandara, Matt Wilbur, Susan Rolandelli, RN, Donna, Trish Low, Jack Hungelmann, Jacqueline Fineblit, Gilbert, Thea Lou Seese, Rosalie, Carol Hilton, Susan Colemen, Don, Ben Petrick, Sandra Howard, Alice Gross, Daniel B. Houston, Rosemary Hunt, Marilyn Berkowitz, Margot Escott, Florence, Andy Stickney, Charles, Michelle Lane, Bob Waite, Ed Stiehle, Nancy, Jim Lammers, Cynthia Entzel, Glen Landenberger, Peggy, Larry Helwig, Dave Carlson, Nancy, Robert Cantor, Roberta, Pam Gehrts, Ann O'Brien, Mariko Ikeda, Kevin M. Peyton, Rees Jenkins, John Wherry, Rudy Molck-Ude, Richard Kramer, Michael Sweeney, Al, Judith R. Post, Gail, Stephen Weisgerber, Keith, Maryann Wolery, Mike Ramsby, Patrick, Steve Waxman, Michael Jacobson, Tim Evensen, Chris Keyser, Seth, Bill, Elizabeth Hammond, John Saldine, Clarence Youngren, Mary Thornhill, Sid, Clare Auble, Janice, Frank Finegan, Jim, Ann, Joy Greenday, Allan Kroland, Kevin and Susan Murray, Paul Almirall, John Wartman, Kimerly Coshow, PhD, Peggy Willocks, Jane Lange, Holly Kroland, Kate Kelsall, Linda, Gene Schelly, Paul Browne, Russ Davidson, Charles Tutt, Wes Tillett, Lori Lynn Jaffe-Brous, Sara Haines, Tom Berdine, Jean Burns, Penny Brown, Linda Rozen, Ruth, Jenny Webster, Betsy, Sean Doody, Gary K. Wooten, Ruth L. Lotzer, Anita Decaro, Patti Lightner, and Karyn Spilberg,

The Parkinson Action Network staff helped to keep me in touch with the real PD world: Joan Samuelson, Laura Jane Cohen, Amy Comstock, Mary Richards, Christy Hahn, and Ben Kirby.

My fellow board members at the Parkinson Association of Minnesota were also very supportive. Thanks to Brooke Bengston, Paul Blom, Jill Breczinski, Kevin Burkart, Ramie Delmoor, Barb Green, Kathy Green, Jerry Kissell, Kris Maser, Leonetta Rence, Eileen Smith, and Sandy Varpness. Also thank you to Rose Wichmann, Joan Gardner, and Catherine Wielinski at the Struthers Parkinson Center.

For their patient listening and intelligent, forthright questions, I thank Lauri Carlson and all of the students in the Jungle and Prairie classrooms: Simran Alter, Tate Bosler, Arlen Bonson-Anderson, Maddie Caruso, Grace Clark, Bennett Christensen, Meara Cline, Nathaniel Danforth, Evan Dunn, Jordan Eckhoff-Bennett, Hunter Franke, Sam Leikind, Angela Leverone, Arius Liuzzi, Ellie Martinson, Laurel Neufeld and Luke Pemberton; Lili Herbert and her advisory group: Jessica Ahlers, Abdul Ali, Isabel Bushway, Alex Christensen, Dave Drevecky, Josh Draves-Kellerman, Ben Gesensway, Talia Glass, Chesa Greene, Matt Jarvis, Theo Mongeau, Caroline Mitchell, Si Nasnan, Eleanor Pearson, Diana Sarmiento, Connor Soles and Sierra Wolff.

A big thanks to B.T., Lee, and Tory at Cities97 and to Moon and Staci at KS95 Radio for providing welcome distractions when I needed them.

John Lofy's friendship, wisdom, encouragement, and excellent professional advice came just when I needed them.

Ali Sands, CMT, massaged away my tension and gave her love and encouragement.

And deep gratitude to Anne Lamott, whom I have never met, but whose writings got me through this, *Bird by Bird*.

Index